ww

ALSO BY INGRID BACCI

The Art of Effortless Living

and published by Bantam Books

Ingrid Bacci, Ph.D.

EFFORTLESS
PAIN
RELIEF

A GUIDE TO SELF-HEALING
FROM CHRONIC PAIN

BANTAM BOOKS

LONDON • TORONTO • SYDNEY • AUCKLAND • JOHANNESBURG

EFFORTLESS PAIN RELIEF
A BANTAM BOOK: 0 553 81735 3

First publication in Great Britain

PRINTING HISTORY
Bantam edition published 2005

1 3 5 7 9 10 8 6 4 2

Designed by Karolina Harris

Bantam Books are published by Transworld Publishers,
61–63 Uxbridge Road, London W5 5SA,
a division of The Random House Group Ltd,
in Australia by Random House Australia (Pty) Ltd,
20 Alfred Street, Milsons Point, Sydney, NSW 2061, Australia,
in New Zealand by Random House New Zealand Ltd,
18 Poland Road, Glenfield, Auckland 10, New Zealand
and in South Africa by Random House (Pty) Ltd,
Endulini, 5a Jubilee Road, Parktown 2193, South Africa.

Printed and bound in Great Britain by
Cox & Wyman Ltd, Reading, Berkshire.

Papers used by Transworld Publishers are natural, recyclable
products made from wood grown in sustainable forests. The
manufacturing processes conform to the environmental
regulations of the country of origin.

For my father, who taught me to think and feel deeply,
and to my mother, who was always there

Acknowledgments

Deepest thanks go to my literary agent and friend, Stephanie Von Hirschberg. Through numerous conversations, she gently prodded me into fine-tuning and systematizing my ideas so as to give birth to this book. Thanks go also to Leslie Meredith, my talented editor at Simon & Schuster. She spared no efforts in polishing and pruning what began as an occasionally verbose manuscript.

Certain colleagues have played a particularly important role in my professional evolution. My experience—as both patient and practitioner—of craniosacral therapy has influenced my perception of the healing process. Thanks go to all the teachers under whom I have studied craniosacral therapy through the Upledger Institute. Special thanks to the institute's founder, Dr. John Upledger, and to Lisa Upledger, who has been both mentor and teacher to me.

I have been fortunate to have a close friend, colleague, and gifted physical therapist in Meryle Richman. Through every step of the evolution of this book, I have shared and discussed my ideas with her and profited from her valuable feedback. When we have had enough of ideas, a good dinner in her company, a thirty-mile bike ride, or a trip to the theater has offered just the right diversion.

I cannot imagine closer friends than Susan and Michael Lanzano. They are my constant emotional and intellectual support team, available for me throughout the writing of this book, as in all aspects of my life. My good friend Beverly Lieberman has also been unwavering in her support, reminding me that I am here to help others heal themselves, as I learned to heal myself.

Our clients are our best teachers. I am particularly grateful to Michael Alfano, Josephine Kovacs, and Anthony Pisacano for having given me the opportunity to work with them.

My family forms my bedrock and foundation. To my mother, my stepmother, Maristella, and my sisters Madeleine, Lavinia, and Donatella (in order of age!), heartfelt gratitude for the love you share so willingly. You are always in my heart.

Contents

PART III: YOUR FEELINGS:
LETTING GO OF EMOTIONAL STRESS

EFFORTLESS PAIN RELIEF

Introduction

If you suffer from chronic pain, you are not alone. Chronic pain is a social and personal problem of epidemic proportions in our society. In the course of their lifetime, 80 percent of Americans will suffer from chronic pain related to dysfunction of the muscles, bones, and joints. In 2004, at least 50 million Americans were living in chronic pain. Back pain is the leading cause of visits to doctors, hospitalization, surgery, and work disability. The Centers for Disease Control and Prevention (CDC) estimated in 2002 that one-third of all Americans had some form of joint disease, most commonly osteoarthritis. And a new musculoskeletal pain syndrome, identified in 1990 as fibromyalgia, has become the second most commonly diagnosed chronic pain disorder after osteoarthritis. By 2004, an estimated 8 million people were said to be suffering from fibromyalgia, 85 percent of them women.

If you suffer from chronic pain related to the bones, joints, or muscles, have not yet found adequate relief, and feel frustrated at the limited assistance available to you, *this book is for you.* It offers you a thorough—and unusually simple—understanding of the causes of chronic neuromuscular, joint, and skeletal pain, along with a clear, step-by-step process for reducing and possibly even eliminating pain. Unfortunately, traditional health care has proven to be woefully inad-

equate for people suffering from chronic pain. Of all physical illnesses and nonacute problems, chronic pain is recognized as the one
least susceptible to treatment with traditional health care techniques,
and according to *The Journal of the American Medical Association*,
pain is the number-one reason people turn to alternative medicine.

Traditional health care has been unable to meet the demand for
effective therapy and unable to stem the growth of chronic pain. The
cost to our society is increasingly burdensome. When we look at standard medical treatments for neuromuscular, skeletal, and joint dys-
functions, we see why. There are two predominant modes of therapy:
surgery and medication. Each of them has significant drawbacks.
Surgery is beneficial in some cases but is not always a viable option.
Moreover, even where surgery is a possible form of treatment, its benefits are far more limited than the public generally believes. A survey
conducted in 2003 by the American Academy of Physical Medicine
and Rehabilitation concluded that a full 48 percent of the population
believes that surgery is the only real cure for at least half of all low-
back-pain cases. But, the academy continued, surgery is actually effective in *less than 5 percent* of cases! In a similar vein, a report
published in 2003 in *The New England Journal of Medicine* said that
doctors are far too aggressive in using operations to treat pain. Finally,
according to a Norwegian study of 126 disk-surgery patients, four
years after surgery those who had been operated on had equivalent
levels of pain to those who had not. The implications are that the ad-
vantages of surgery are more limited than we tend to think and that
anyone with chronic pain should seriously consider other options before going under the knife.

The second standard form of medical treatment for chronic pain is
medication. Its goal is usually either to reduce inflammation or to
suppress symptoms. It is most useful as a short-term therapy. Over the
long term, however, it can result in toxic side effects, sometimes even
including severe intestinal bleeding and heart disease. Patients on regular medication can also expect, as the months and years go by, to
need increasing doses of such drugs, which may harm their health
and which treat only the symptoms and not the source of their dis-

comfort. They are likely to experience a gradual increase of pain and disability; anxiety over a physical condition that seems beyond their control; a sense of powerlessness; and the depressing feeling that they must live with a problem that is incurable.

While medication tends to represent the road most taken, research indicates that it can sometimes be less effective than other less expensive but more intensive and empowering therapies. For example, the U.S. Headache Consortium, led by the American Academy of Neurology, recommends relaxation training—including meditation and progressive muscle relaxation—over drug therapy as the therapy of choice in dealing with migraines.

Obviously, something is missing from the standard diagnosis of the *causes* of pain. That diagnosis usually seeks the origin of pain in a structural or biochemical imbalance. Yet the underlying cause of pain is in most cases neither structural nor biochemical. Once you understand the true causes of chronic pain, you will be able to find effective solutions that you yourself can apply to reducing your own pain, empowering yourself, and finding a better lifestyle.

When you suffer from chronic pain, you must look "outside the box" to find innovative, accurate, objective, and—once understood—*obvious* answers. The solutions offered in this book show you how you can become your own best doctor. Along the way, you will also free yourself from excessive reliance on medical and insurance options that become increasingly expensive and drain your pocketbook even as they provide mixed results.

The highlights of *Effortless Pain Relief* include these revelations about the fundamental causes of and solutions for chronic pain.

1. *The most common cause of chronic pain is neither structural nor biochemical imbalances, but rather lifestyle habits.* What causes chronic pain? In a few cases, genetic predisposition or physical trauma endured through accidents plays a role. However—more important by far—in a full 80 percent of cases, the single most critical factor in the development of chronic pain is lifestyle habits. In fact, even if your pain started with an accident or has a genetic basis, it is

often the lifestyle habits that you have developed to accommodate to the pain that bear primary responsibility for your pain.

"Lifestyle habits," as the term is used here, are the unconscious habits that involve the way you live in your body: the way you breathe, stand, and move; and the way you store physical and emotional stress in your tissues. Over months and years, these unconscious habits foster increasing physical stress, eventually wearing down muscles, joints, and bones, thus causing escalating discomfort. You can be your own worst enemy, and your own lifestyle habits can be the cause of your dis-ease. But knowing this also has very positive implications. Just as developing unconscious habits of body and mind can result in pain, so too becoming conscious of these habits and altering them can alleviate and even eliminate pain. Rather than having to rely on outside sources to help you, you will discover that *you* are your best resource for reducing and even eliminating chronic pain. This simple fact makes *Effortless Pain Relief* the first and only complete guide to the self-empowering process of healing from chronic pain. It shows you exactly how and why the way you live in your body may have created the pain from which you suffer. It also shows you how and why changing the way you live in your body frees you from pain. Finally, it offers you a complete tool kit for implementing that process.

2. *Lifestyle habits that create pain are both the expression and the cause of stress.* In the course of a lifetime, we experience many forms of stress. Stress can be physical (for example, an injury or repetitive stress syndrome), mental (for example, excessive work demands), or emotional (for example, ongoing anxiety). No matter what the origin of stress, however, it is always reflected in the body. Like physical stress, mental and emotional stresses are acted out through changes at all levels of the body: biochemical, neurological, and physiological. All chronic stresses also reflect themselves in certain physical habits, or ways of experiencing and responding with your body. These habits involve unnecessary physical tensions. The tensions of lifestyle habits contribute to pain, pain creates further stress, stress creates further

tension, which contributes to further pain, and so on. By understanding the many aspects of stress, how it is reflected in lifestyle habits, and how these habits create tension and discomfort in the body, you will also begin to understand how to reverse the stress and lifestyle habits that underlie your problem and reduce your pain.

3. Body awareness is the primary vehicle for changing the lifestyle habits that express and create stress and pain. Just as pain is a physical experience in your body, so too the stresses and lifestyle habits that create physical pain are experiences of your body. You can reduce your pain by becoming conscious of bodily patterns and experiences that are unconscious and by changing those bodily patterns and experiences. For example, you can reduce your pain by changing the way you breathe under stress, the way you sit at the computer, the way you walk down the street, the way you react with tension when someone challenges you, or the way you feel anxiety on a visceral level when you are under internal or external pressure.

You can reduce your pain by changing your body. This does *not* mean that your pain will improve as a result of your doing physical exercise. Physical exercise can be a very useful adjunct to the process of healing from chronic pain, but there are already many books available on that subject and exercise is not the best method of healing chronic pain. The best way you can heal is by *becoming aware of the way you live in your body and changing it*: the way you respond to situations, the way you move, the way you react to pressures around you. Healing results from heightened body awareness, and this book shows you how to develop that awareness. As you develop body awareness, you will automatically know how to release unconscious tensions that foster pain.

4. Your body teaches you how to heal from chronic pain. As you work with this book, you will explore and experience your body more fully. By enhancing your awareness of your body—of how it feels moment by moment, how it functions, how it reacts to situations, and how it stores your personal history—you will naturally and organically begin to learn things about your body and about yourself that you did not know. In this process, you will shift the way you live in your body, adopting patterns that reduce discomfort and increase ease, while enlarging your overall sense of well-being.

The body is a teacher. If you listen to it, you can learn from it. You will learn to listen to your body's signals. Just as emotional pain in a personal relationship can be an indication of poor communication between partners, so too, when you are in physical pain, your body may be signaling to you that you are doing something that is causing a problem. If you fail to pick up on the meaning of that signal, your discomfort may become habitual. In the chapters that follow, you will discover what it means to pick up on and respond effectively to your body's signals.

Some of the body's signals are purely physical. For example, you may lean your head too far forward when you sit for hours at the computer. This will eventually give you a headache, neck pain, or temporomandibular joint (TMJ) problems, or shoulder trouble. In this case, a physical habit of poor posture is creating pain. Yet a great many signals you receive from your body are not solely physical. They have a mental or emotional component as well because the body holds our mental and emotional stresses. These stresses—some of which are conscious but many of which are unconscious—are recorded as subtle body shifts and tensions, which, if held over a long period of time, cause physical distress.

We experience and express our emotions in and through our bodies. We are aware of this every time we feel our stomach flutter when we face a challenging situation: we experience a tightening of the chest or jaw in anger; or we feel our neck or shoulders tense in anticipation of a deadline. Long-term mental and emotional stresses leave their mark in the body's physiology and can contribute to your pain. As you become more aware of your body, you will also become more aware of the mental and emotional stresses that register themselves in your body and contribute to chronic pain.

5. *Healing chronic physical pain can involve both your mind and your heart.* All forms of stress, whether mental, emotional, or physical in origin, express themselves through unconscious habits of physical tension in the body. As you learn to release physical tension habits through heightened body awareness, you will simultaneously reap emotional and mental benefits: You will reduce mental and emotional stress. You may also become aware of mental and emotional attitudes that contribute to your pain. You may decide to let go of some of these attitudes. All aspects of our lives intersect in our bodies, and healing the body can create deep ripples of change in the type of person you want to be and how you choose to interface with the world.

6. *Stress is associated with feelings of disempowerment, and disempowerment is often an ingredient in the development of chronic pain.* When stressed, we feel controlled by something outside ourselves. An accident, a sudden illness, getting fired, or losing money in a stock market slide are obviously stressful, yet life also presents us with many subtler stresses: a temperamental family member who always has to be right; a rigid work environment or difficult colleagues; long commutes; a hypervigilant superego that criticizes us constantly. Much of life can feel beyond our control. When it does, we feel disempowered to some degree. Stress and feelings of disempowerment tend to go together.

The most obvious emotions that stem from a sense of disempowerment are chronic anger or frustration and chronic anxiety or fear. *Effortless Pain Relief* shows you how these feelings manifest as physical reactions of stress and how these stress reactions create pain. It also shows you how to use your body awareness to let go of negative emotions of fear and anger to reduce stress, become more empowered, and eliminate chronic pain. Once you see the intimate relationship among chronic pain, stress, and feelings of disempowerment, you will have a road map for healing your physical pain. In the process, you will develop greater control over your own life.

My Journey Out of Pain

This book offers a unique pathway to healing from chronic pain, a pathway that takes you into a deeper experience and appreciation of your body, its messages, tools, and response patterns. I know this approach works because it is how I overcame my own crippling pain and because I have taught it to others so that they could do the same.

I have worked for years to understand and resolve the problem of chronic pain, both for myself and for my patients. Today I work as an alternative health care practitioner specializing in movement therapy and in a manual approach to bodywork called craniosacral therapy. In addition to my private practice, I teach pain reduction seminars at hospitals and HMOs, teach craniosacral therapy nationally, run retreats, write books and articles, and create audio programs and videos on reducing stress and pain. At the age of fifty-nine, I am graced with radiant health. I run, bike, swim, hike, practice yoga almost daily, and enjoy intensive circuit training workouts. But I wasn't always so healthy. Nor has my professional work always been in alternative health care. I entered that field after leaving a career as a college professor and in the process of working through fifteen years of disabling pain. My journey into personal healing, combined with training in several approaches to bodywork, and my twenty years in private practice helping others heal from chronic pain have led me to the approach described in this book. It is an approach that works.

I was born in New York City, the daughter of well-established, first-generation European immigrants. My father was an internationally renowned mathematician, who was frequently invited to teach abroad. My mother was a literary editor, homemaker, and wonderful mom. By the time my twin sister and I were nine, we had lived in Europe for several years and, in addition to English, spoke French and Italian fluently. Then we moved back to New York City and my parents got divorced.

I was privileged to receive the very best that education can offer, at the Brearley School, a private girls' school with an outstanding reputation. On completing high school, I attended Radcliffe College, the sister of Harvard University, which merged with Harvard in 1977. I graduated in 1967 first in my class and with highest honors, then went to England to study on a fellowship at Cambridge University. On my return to the United States, I completed a doctorate in philosophy at Columbia University, then became an assistant professor of Philosophy at the State University of New York. My life seemed to be running smoothly and successfully.

But within five years, everything had changed. Over a period of a few months, my strength disappeared and my body inexplicably collapsed. I developed excruciating low back pain and began to have burning sensations throughout my body. When bed rest didn't solve the problem, I began to seek medical advice. I was hospitalized twice in New York City's finest hospitals, subjected to endless tests, and given numerous anti-inflammatories, painkillers, and mood elevators. I visited every doctor I could imagine: neurologists, orthopedists, internists, and rheumatologists. I also tried chiropractors, massage therapists, physical therapists, and nutritionists. I was given no conclusive diagnosis, other than that I seemed to be suffering from a collagen disease. Today, I would have been told I had a severe case of fibromyalgia and of chronic fatigue syndrome. None of the remedies did much more than offer symptomatic relief. After fruitless and time-consuming forays in a number of directions, I was finally told that I would just have to live with my condition.

I went on extensive sick leave from university teaching. I had no other choice. I spent three years in and out of bed, but mostly in bed. On a good day I could take a short walk around the block of my New York City apartment, always with a family member or friend to guide and support me. On a bad day I was confined to my room, an inmate in prison, my indeterminate sentence stretching out darkly before me. I suffered from extreme loneliness, severe anxiety, and deep depression. Life seemed hopeless. The best experts had been unable to help me, and I was unable to help myself.

After three years of growing hopelessness and despair, one day I came across an article about a woman named Elsa Gindler, who had lived in the early part of the twentieth century. As a young woman she had been confined in a sanatorium with severe tuberculosis. She had been told that there was little hope for her recovery. Gindler cured herself, however, through a process of becoming more and more deeply aware of her breathing. Her growing awareness enabled her to change her breathing patterns in a way that helped her body heal. Elsa Gindler later became famous for establishing a form of self-awareness training and self-healing called Sensory Awareness. That approach achieved popularity in the United States primarily through the work of Gindler's student and associate Charlotte Selver.

Reading about Elsa Gindler offered me my first ray of hope in years. Here was something to inspire me and lift me out of my gloom. Like me, Gindler had been told there was little chance of her healing, yet she had healed herself by following an approach that had never occurred to me: observing and experimenting with her own bodily sensations, gradually learning how to gain control over them and to change them in a way that cured her disease.

Since no one had been able to help me, I decided to try to help myself. I began to work with my breathing. I observed it, noticed when it felt more or less restricted, and slowly, painstakingly, found my way to deepening and relaxing it.

As I worked with changing my breathing patterns, it became quite clear that the way I breathed affected my level of pain. When I breathed more deeply, easily, and calmly, my pain would gradually diminish.

Through this form of bodily self-awareness, I learned a great deal about myself. Most especially I recognized that the stresses of my life always translated into my breathing patterns and that, if I could shift my breathing, I could decrease my stress, which seemed in turn to reduce my pain. In addition, I began to sense that I could become aware of how I used my arms, my legs, my torso, my muscles in general, this process might also lead to a reduction in pain. But I didn't know how to proceed.

A friend opened the door for me when she recommended Alexander Technique training, a form of movement therapy that uses your own senses to relax the body, reduce chronic pain and tension, and improve the body's alignment. (Some of the core principles of the Alexander Technique are described in chapters 6 and 7). My first lesson in the Alexander Technique, a mere thirty minutes, gave me such a feeling of well-being that I decided on the spot to study it. Three years later, I was a certified teacher and I was also feeling a lot better, having learned to let go of many of the unconscious habits of tension and effort that had contributed to my pain.

I resigned from my academic career and opened a private practice in the Alexander Technique. Although I was feeling much better and had begun to teach, I still suffered bouts of pain and was constantly stiff and frequently sore. Since enhanced body awareness had helped me a great deal, I wanted to continue exploring that pathway and resolved to study other systems, including Feldenkrais Awareness Through Movement, Somatics, and Aston Patterning. All these disciplines invite you into the body, increasing your presence to yourself as well as your ability to perceive, respond to, and master the way your body deals with life's events. The essence of these teachings (described primarily in chapters 8 and 9) is simple: reduce the effort you expend by paying very close attention to how you move and what muscles you use in movement, and you will enhance the fluidity, grace, and ease of your body.

Slowing down and observing my body helped me see more clearly into my body, its problems, and how to conquer those problems. I spent hours on the floor exploring tiny movements, learning how to make them slowly, softly, and gently. I was gradually undoing the knots created by years of stressful living piled on top of a genetically inherited physical structure that suffered from scoliosis and other misalignments. I learned that one of the fastest routes to letting go of chronic pain is to focus on learning how to reduce effort, to make a discipline of exploring effortlessness.

The more I studied how to decrease effort in my life, the more my pain receded. The more I taught this art, the more my clients' pain diminished. By now most of my clients were people who, like me, had explored traditional therapies and found them limited. They needed help, and they were willing to look in out-of-the-way places. I was glad to assist them.

The next step in my own healing process came with the discovery that the more present I became to my physical body and the more I was able to reduce my physical tensions, the more present I also became to emotions that were unconsciously contributing to my pain. Part of this discovery happened as a natural result of my increasing awareness of my own body. Part of it happened as a result of exploring craniosacral therapy, a powerful hands-on treatment that helps release deep adhesions and tissue tensions from the body and that in the process often evokes emotions and memories that have contributed to the creation of those tensions. (The story of how emotions translate into pain, and how to release emotions that create pain, forms the subject of chapters 10 through 15.)

I also trained and became certified in craniosacral therapy, which I now integrate into the movement work I do with my clients. I also teach it nationally to doctors, physical therapists, chiropractors, massage therapists, and occupational therapists through the Upledger Institute, one of the world's leading centers for craniosacral therapy.

I discovered that the combination of body and movement awareness work, along with gentle hands-on therapies such as craniosacral therapy, creates a synergy that motivates the deepest layers of healing, whether the origins of that healing lie in physical or in emotional pain.

Out of necessity, I became a pioneer in my own healing. Fifteen years after I started my journey, I was not only older and wiser but also completely free of pain and able to engage in any sport or activity I desired. In my early thirties, I had felt like a ninety-year-old inmate of a nursing home. In my fifties, I feel and—according to others—look like a thirty-year-old athlete. The odds were against this. Yet I believe that my path has not been unusual and that my life has blessed me with a learning that I am meant to share with others who suffer from chronic pain, so that they too can let go of what doesn't serve them through becoming more aware of how to live gracefully, easily, and powerfully in their bodies.

Today, I am a pioneer in helping others heal. I have helped thousands of people who have come to work with me, many of whom knocked on my door out of desperation that nothing else had helped. The lectures, seminars, books, articles, videos, and audio programs I have created all have one purpose: to introduce you to a process of self-healing that is simple and obvious in its core, yet that most of us overlook. Though I have put my own words to that process, the fundamental ideas I express in this book are not new. Like any ideas that work, they have been discovered and rediscovered again and again. In the pages that follow, I invite you to take the time first to understand the origins of your pain and then to follow the step-by-step process of reducing your pain. You are going to find this process very pleasurable. Enjoy it!

Part I

WHAT'S CAUSING YOUR PAIN?

1

PICTURES OF PAIN AND HEALING

To heal from chronic pain, you have an abundance of options. Each specialist who sees you is likely to praise the virtues of his or her approach and may discount the value of other therapies. Chances are that if you are not professionally involved in medicine or alternative therapies, you will have a difficult time trying to figure out what avenue to pursue and why.

You need to find out as soon as possible what is causing your pain. Then you can begin to consider what therapies might be most useful. Stress, in the form of neuromuscular tension, is a leading cause of pain, which results from lifestyle habits that we adopt in the course of handling the pressures of our lives. Consequently, treating pain requires you to change these physical, mental, and emotional lifestyle habits and to reverse their cumulative effect.

The case studies below show how, by reversing certain lifestyle habits, four of my clients reduced their physical pain.

MELISSA

Melissa was forty-eight years old when she first sought my professional assistance. She had been suffering from bouts of chronic pain for eight years. Her symptoms included low back and hip pain, as well as shoulder and neck tension that sometimes escalated into debilitating headaches. Melissa had been told she had fibromyalgia.

The term "fibromyalgia" formally entered the medical lexicon in 1990 as a result of doctors' having been flooded over a number of years with cases of chronic pain that defied medical diagnosis. Research identifying these patients' common traits led to the definition of a fibromyalgia syndrome. Patients are deemed to suffer from fibromyalgia when they feel pain in response to pressure on at least eleven of eighteen "tender points" on the body, points where muscle tendon and ligaments attach to bone. Since 1997, fibromyalgia has become one of the most commonly diagnosed musculoskeletal disorders. There is no known biochemical cause of fibromyalgia, and standard tests, such as X-rays, myelograms, CAT scans and MRIs, fail to isolate specific structural origins of the syndrome. This is not surprising, since the label "fibromyalgia" is actually a blanket term covering a wide variety of pain disorders that have their origin in soft-tissue lesions, adhesions, strains, and imbalances, most of which are not picked up by the usual tests. Once the soft tissue of muscles and connective tissue is damaged, that damage can cause pain in locally affected areas and can also spread throughout the entire body, along the weblike structure of connective tissue that envelops and supports all the body's organs and tissues.

Like many persons diagnosed with fibromyalgia, Melissa had been given medication to manage her pain. She had also been told she would simply have to cope with this problem, for which there was no known cure. Melissa was given no guidance in understanding either how her pain syndrome had developed or how she might reverse some of its effects. Naturally enough, she felt depressed and defeated by the diagnosis. A growing sense of powerlessness about her body cast a pall over her life.

I suspected that Melissa's pain syndrome was not purely structural or biochemical in origin and was interested in finding out more about her in order to get to the bottom of her situation. During our first few sessions, Melissa told me some of the details of her personal life. She had had a difficult childhood under the care of a narcissistic mother,

had married and eventually divorced a successful but alcoholic businessman, was the mother of two children, and had herself pursued a
hard-driving though erratic career. Her life had had its share of stress,
and the combination of her illness and ongoing personal and professional demands continued to put her under daily pressure. I was sure
that the origin of Melissa's pain lay in the way she was living in her
body, day after day, month after month, and year after year. Something she was doing with her body was causing it to underfunction. If
we could change that, she would feel better.

We began our work together by exploring and making changes in
some of her deep-seated physical habits. We started by having Melissa
focus on one of her most important physical habits: the way she
breathed. Her job was simply to become aware of how she breathed
under everyday circumstances. I gave her some guidelines for evaluating her breathing patterns, which I'll give you later in this book.
When she applied these guidelines, she was surprised to discover that
her breathing was relatively uneven, shallow, and somewhat labored.
In addition, she frequently held her breath. This pattern of constricted breathing might have been contributing to her physical pain.
Constricted breathing deprives the muscles of the vital oxygen that
keeps them healthy and also often corresponds to neuromuscular tension in the body. If we could open up Melissa's breathing, we would
be reducing her muscle tension and oxygenating her tissues.

Melissa learned some breathing exercises to help her slow down
her breathing, deepen it, and make it more regular. I also asked her to
become aware of when she held her breath and to try to replace this
habit with more even breathing. Melissa worked on becoming conscious of her breathing and applying the new breathing style throughout her daily activities. She noticed that the more she focused on
breathing deeply and evenly, the less her back and hip pain bothered
her and the less she suffered from headaches.

Now Melissa felt the effectiveness of my approach to reducing
pain through changing physical habits. As she continued to work on
breath awareness, we also explored other physical habits that will be
described later in this book. Like her breathing patterns, these habits

were unconscious, and, also like her breathing patterns, they contributed to her discomfort by creating or exacerbating neuromuscular tension. By the time Melissa and I stopped working together, her pain of eight years' duration was 70 percent improved, and she had the information and techniques to continue making progress on her own. Today, her pain has virtually disappeared.

Let's compare Melissa's course of mind-body therapy with traditional treatments for chronic pain to see why Melissa had found no pain relief from the standard medical treatments. When surgery is not an option—as in Melissa's case—remedies for chronic pain tend to include the use of medication, physical manipulation, prescribed exercises, or some combination of these. A doctor prescribes medication; a chiropractor, physical therapist, massage therapist, or other body worker applies manual therapy; and a physical therapist, sometimes in collaboration with an orthopedist, prescribes exercises. Patients who receive medication or manual therapy tend to play a passive role in their own treatment. They may not be asked to observe or change lifestyle habits that involve the way they live in their body. Even when professionals treating them recognize such habits as a concern, these professionals may not possess either adequate time to retrain their clients or professional training in sophisticated skills that are required to help patients change deep-seated, largely unconscious habits of physical stress.

Patients who work with exercises to reduce their pain take a more active role. They embark on a course of action to make changes in their own bodies. Yet even these patients do not on the whole address their daily habits of body use or look at their lifestyle habits in anything more than a cursory manner. Such habits inevitably play an important role in the origin and chronic nature of patients' pain, since pain usually involves structural and functional imbalances that have developed over a period of time. If lifestyle habits underlie patients' pain, the benefits of medication and manipulation are likely to be limited. Specific exercises may be useful, but if they fail to address the physical tension that causes pain, they too will have only limited effect. Exercises would be more effective if they were taught in conjunction with a therapy program focused on correcting long-term dysfunctional tension habits involving posture, movement, and chronic stress.

In Melissa's case, medication, manipulation, and exercise had failed to help her in the past and were not likely to work in the future without an additional approach. A key physical habit—namely, the way Melissa breathed—played an important role in her pain syndrome, and by changing this physical habit she released deep levels of neuromuscular tension and eased her pain, which was largely due to excess muscular stress.

Melissa noticed that the breathing work not only lessened her physical discomfort, it also reduced her anxiety and improved her mental focus. A simple physical technique—breath awareness combined with deep, relaxed breathing—enhanced her physiological, mental, and emotional functioning. Melissa's mental state, her emotional state, and her physical state were all connected; when one improved, the others improved as well.

When you change a way you live in your body, other mental and emotional changes result. Pain is a *whole-body phenomenon*, the consequence of a subtle interaction of our physiology with our hearts and minds. So too is healing.

MIKE

An elderly gentleman named Mike came to me with chronic low-grade back pain. His pain had begun gradually in middle age, worsening progressively until he found it difficult to stand for any length of time. Mike avoided lines in grocery stores and at bus stops, and when he attended receptions or dinner parties, he sought out a chair so that he could sit rather than stand while chatting with other guests. I asked Mike to walk around the room and then come to a stop. I noticed that when he stopped and stood, he locked his knees. When we lock our knees—bringing them back as far as they will go rather than bending them slightly and keeping them "soft"—this causes the pelvis to drop forward, so that it no longer supports the spine above it. As a result, the back becomes swayed. When the back sways, the muscles of the lumbar area have to brace in an effort to stabilize the spine. Over time this bracing reaction overworks and stresses the muscles of the low back, which become increasingly contracted, contributing to discomfort, muscle spasms, and even herniated discs or arthritis.

I showed Mike how to release the pressure on his back by unlocking his knees, and I sent him away with instructions to notice when he locked his knees and to unlock them whenever possible.

A week later, Mike was back in my office, eager to share his observations. He had discovered, to his surprise, that he locked his knees almost constantly. He had never noticed this before. He also noticed that when he paid attention to unlocking his knees, this greatly relieved his back pain. Mike's habit of knee locking created neuromuscular tension. By becoming conscious of and changing that habit—the way he stood—he had eliminated excess tension in his low back muscles.

Mike shared some further insights. When he locked his knees, his body seemed to brace, becoming rigid and inflexible. When he unlocked his knees, his body was softer and more pliable, less like a stiff rod and more like a strong young sapling swaying in the wind. Keeping his knees unlocked gave him a better sense of balance, flexibility, and flow. Although this feeling was physical, it also affected his mental and emotional mood. When his knees were locked, he felt psychologically and physically rigid, brittle, and unbending, as if he needed to defend himself. With his knees unlocked, he felt more in control but less controlling. Mike wondered whether he had gotten into the habit of locking his knees as a defensive, self-protective posture. Whether or not this was the case, he noticed that by becoming more conscious of his body and releasing his physical habit of locking, he decreased his physical pain while increasing his sense of mental and emotional well-being. He was more relaxed. Mike realized that his physical, mental, and emotional states were interrelated: physical tension seemed to be tied to mental and emotional tension, and physical ease was connected to mental and emotional ease.

Our mental, emotional, and physical states do not exist separately and apart from each other. Becoming more conscious of how to influence our physical bodies can have a salutary effect on our mental and emotional lives. Similarly, mental and emotional states can affect our physiology. As we shall see, this chain of mutual influences has significant implications for treating and eliminating chronic pain.

When Mike felt the emotional and mental improvements that came from making a physical change in his body stance, he discovered for himself the ancient wisdom that is embedded in the philosophy and practice of Eastern spiritual practices such as chi gung, tai chi, and yoga. These practices have their foundation in body awareness and self-mastery. They recognize that the body's sensations offer important information about our well-being. They focus on improving our total state of well-being by improving our presence to the body. They recognize that the more we focus on developing skills that increase our grace, suppleness, physical ease, and physical self-awareness, the more we feel physically healthy and mentally and emotionally supple and empowered.

The wisdom of these ancient arts and my own personal and professional experience of working with clients in chronic pain serve as a foundation for the approach to chronic pain reduction in this book. My approach emphasizes, first, that habits of body use are the primary cause of physical pain; second, that these bodily habits cause pain because they foster excessive neuromuscular tension; third, that enhancing bodily self-awareness is the critical component for healing the neuromuscular tension that creates chronic pain; and fourth, that the practice of bodily awareness shows us how to reduce physical, mental, and emotional stresses that contribute to our neuromuscular tension and pain.

Mike and Melissa reduced their chronic pain by becoming aware of physical habits that involved unconscious muscular tensions and learning how to release them. Melissa did this by relaxing her whole body through breath awareness. Mike reduced unconscious tensions by improving his body alignment. Mike and Melissa did not improve because a doctor or therapist did something to them. They improved because they changed something in themselves. Their stories demonstrate that exploring how we live in our bodies can be a powerful way to heal from physical pain.

CLARA

In the process of looking at and altering habits of body use, we sometimes make surprising discoveries about ourselves, discoveries that extend beyond simple physical realizations into insights about our personalities and about how our personalities affect our experience of pain. A thirty-five-year-old woman named Clara was referred to me as a result of numbness in her legs that did not respond to conventional treatments. When I examined Clara, I discovered a high level of tension in the pelvic region. Nerves, arteries, and veins pass through the pelvis to the legs. Constriction of any one of these as a consequence of pelvic tension can result in numbness in the legs. Tension in the pelvic muscles can also put excess strain on the muscles of the legs, restricting nerve function and circulation in those areas.

Like Mike's and Melissa's, Clara's problems seemed to be related to excess muscle and pelvic tension. Clara said that she could not herself feel this tension. This was not surprising, as her numbness indicated that she had trouble feeling her body. Lack of feeling is frequently a consequence of excess tension. My challenge was to help Clara approach her body in such a way that she reduced that tension. Clara agreed to follow my recommendations, and over several sessions, during which she lay at ease on a bodywork table, I had her focus on simply feeling and appreciating the sensation of her pelvis. I told her neither to expect particular sensations nor to try to relax her pelvis. Her only goal was to feel whatever her pelvis felt like. Since tension is related to loss of feeling, improving Clara's ability to feel would in turn reduce her physical tension. This is what happened, and along the way, Clara had an illumining realization. She discovered she was uncomfortable with feeling herself. She wanted to interfere with her sensations: to react to, suppress, interpret, do something about, or in some other way control the feelings going on in her body.

Clara's situation is not uncommon. How often have you popped an Advil or an Aleve, rather than feel physical discomfort? We often try to avoid physical sensations that we think are unpleasant. We do the same with sensations that involve our emotions, heading for the freezer in search of ice cream or to the cupboard for a box of cookies when a conversation gets too heated and raises feelings we'd rather not address. How often have you denied you felt anger or grief when you thought you weren't supposed to feel it? In all these situations, we use some tactic to control how we feel physically or emotionally rather than allow ourselves to feel what we feel. When we try to control our feelings—physical or emotional—we suppress them. This creates tension, which in turn creates pain.

Clara related to her body as something alien that she needed to control. Unconsciously, she viewed her physical sensations as suspect and problematic. This attitude created tension and confirmed her fears by triggering physical problems. Clara's real problem was her attitude of suspicion and fear toward her own sensations. We have evolved our physical sensations, including sensations of discomfort, as part of feedback that is meant to guide us in surviving and thriving. If we suppress the feedback process, we sabotage nature's intelligence. Clara had become so alienated from her own body that when first asked to explore her physical sensations, she felt she couldn't. She had suppressed her ability to feel behind a wall of tension. As she continued to explore feeling, however, that wall began to dissolve, and then she encountered anxiety and discomfort: feeling itself was uncomfortable. As she learned not to give in to her reactions of anxiety and discomfort, the tension and pain in her body gradually dissipated. She gave up trying to control her body, and her body started feeling better.

Clara came to the realization that her numbness was the consequence of deep-seated tension and her tension resulted from trying to manage and control her feelings and sensations, rather than simply experiencing and accepting them. Her physical numbness and pain had a physical source in neuromuscular tension. Yet that physical tension was also the consequence of mental and emotional attitudes that emphasized her need to control. Clara began to see that letting go might be a better choice than controlling. She improved physically while also discovering healthier emotional and mental options.

Like both Melissa and Mike, Clara reduced her physical pain by exploring and gradually changing a physical habit that was creating tension in her body. All three reduced their physical tension with a self-directed intervention that gave them heightened bodily self-awareness. All three began to observe subtle connections between their physical, mental, and emotional states, connections that indicated that physical pain is often a whole-body expression of interactions between these states. Relaxing into feeling her body helped Clara address and let go of an emotional need to control, which was one cause of her physical discomfort. She became aware of her emotional control issues not through verbal processing but through listening to her body and observing herself more closely. Exploring her ability to feel her body yielded emotional insight that in turn helped her reduce her physical pain.

JEAN

Though we may use physical techniques to alleviate our physical pain, a primary cause of that pain may lie in emotional issues that have an impact on the body. A young woman came to visit me complaining of shoulder pain, from which she had been suffering for three months. Jean was irritated with herself and with her shoulder. As with my other clients, I focused first on helping Jean let go of stress and achieve a deeper state of relaxation through the use of bodily self-awareness techniques that reduced physical tension. I then encouraged her to feel the pain in her shoulder *without resistance*. Rather than reacting to her pain with upset, annoyance, or anger, she was simply to accept, appreciate, and feel the sensations. As she simply explored and observed her physical sensations, her nonjudgmental, nonreactive stance would help her eliminate tension and identify the underlying causes of that tension.

I asked Jean to consider her sensations of pain not as uninvited intruders but rather as a part of herself that was trying to share important information. At first she felt uncomfortable and skittish about this, but after a period of silence, during which she tried to focus on being present to her sensations of pain without judgment, she began to cry. She reported that she was neither crying *from* her physical pain, nor was she crying *about* her physical pain. Her tears were about *another* pain: the death of her mother a few months before Jean's shoulder injury had occurred. Surprisingly to Jean, as she cried out her grief, her shoulder pain eased. Clearly, her physical tension and pain had been connected to emotional tension and pain. After her cry, Jean told me that the pressure of work and family obligations had been such that she had never allowed herself fully to grieve for her mother's parting. She had bottled up her feelings, which had somehow found their way into her shoulder.

A week later, Jean telephoned to tell me that her pain was completely gone. She had devoted much of the week to communing with her mother's spirit and completing her good-byes. We marveled together at the mystery of life and at the fact that a physical discomfort had been her body's way of telling her that she had unfinished emotional business. Jean recognized that her emotional realizations had come not from talking about her mother but through feeling her body. Her grief had been stored far from her conscious mind, in her body's tissues, and physical self-awareness had unlocked emotional self-awareness.

Jean changed the way in which she was relating to her body. She stopped being irritated or angry with her body and complaining about its limitations. She just let it feel the way it felt. She changed a deep-seated habit of judgmentalism, which had surprising results: it reduced both her physical and emotional pain, which had been locked in her tense, contracted tissues.

RECOMMENDATIONS

In the cases of Melissa, Mike, Clara, and Jean, the ultimate physical source of pain was excess neuromuscular and connective tissue stress and tension. In each case, this tension was related to unconscious bodily habits that were released once the patients became aware of them. In each case, the patient's physiological healing was triggered by his or her own actions. And all of them became aware that changing bodily habits improved their mental and emotional state and that mental and emotional attitudes had contributed to their physical pain.

Letting go of chronic pain involves becoming aware of the way you live in, respond, and react to your body and changing it. Your body is not an alien force; it holds the keys to your health. If you learn how to listen to it, work with it, and understand it, you can heal.

The primary source of neuromuscular tension is stress. The word "stress" is a part of our everyday language, but its actual nature is poorly understood. How does stress work its way through the body? What is physical stress? What is emotional stress? What is mental stress? How are these related to one another and how do they contribute to pain? Chapters 2 and 3 will answer these questions.

Once you understand how stress manifests as neuromuscular tension and creates pain, you can learn body awareness techniques and discover how to use them to eliminate the stress that creates pain. You will also be able use these tools to identify and release whatever unique physical, mental, and emotional stresses may underlie your own history of chronic pain. These methods form the subject of chapters 4 through 15.

2

How Stress Creates Pain

Since stress is a primary cause of pain, you need to learn how you can become the principal agent of your own physical improvement and healing. You can start by looking at simple daily situations that create stress in your life.

Negative Emotions, Physical Tension, and the Startle Reflex

Have you ever noticed the feelings you get from watching a particularly upsetting news broadcast on TV: details of a recent terrorist attack; a bad slide on the stock market; fraud and corruption in the corporate world; recent discoveries of unknown health hazards; devastating tornadoes, forest fires, or floods? Events such as these give rise to feelings that are more than mental—they are *physical sensations*. You may feel anger or fear as a knot in your chest or gut. Or you may tense your neck, tighten your shoulders, grip in your thighs, hold your breath, and clench your teeth. Negative emotions such as anger, irritation, fear, and anxiety trigger physical stress in the body, and we tighten up.

On the other hand, positive feelings—such as peace and contentment—express themselves physically as release and expansion. Think of how you feel when you're lying on the beach or floating in warm water on a lazy summer's day, without a care in the world. Chances are you feel open, soft, released, and relaxed. Positive feelings of ease and contentment help you let go physically and enhance bodily freedom and flow.

Negative emotions such as anger and fear are emotional stresses that translate directly into physical neuromuscular tension, a key part of the startle reflex, commonly known as the fight-or-flight response. Triggered by the perception of a threat, the startle reflex plays a major role in the development of chronic pain. In more primitive times, the fight-or-flight response might have been activated by the sight of a tiger or a venomous snake. Today, that same reflex is more likely to kick in when we barely escape colliding with a swerving car on the highway, get fired or get into a confrontation or conflict at work, miss a crucial deadline, or hear that we—or someone close to us—have just been diagnosed with a terminal illness. Distressing events startle us, and we clench.

The startle reflex, along with the negative emotions that accompany and evoke it, also becomes activated in less dramatic ways, by the constant daily pressures of modern living: too many traffic jams for too many days in a row; the relentless pace of work and an overly competitive spirit at the office; medical bills that are too high and insurance payments that are too low; ongoing problems with family members who have health issues; our own health problems; stresses with schools over the education of our children; phone calls from acquaintances who won't stop talking; and just plain too much to do.

Each of us also has a unique personal history that predisposes us to react to specific conditions. For example, if a parent criticized you unduly as a child, as an adult you might be particularly sensitive to criticism and might react to it swiftly, tearfully, or angrily. Or if you were physically attacked years ago in a wooded area, even today you might be unable to walk through the woods without a feeling of unaccountable dread.

When we perceive a threat and the startle reflex turns on, our emotional and physical reactions are so commingled that they are indistinguishable. Negative emotions *are* physical tensions. We register a conscious feeling of fear or anger as a physical reaction that can include tension in our diaphragm; shallow, tight breathing; and gripping sensations in the neck, chest, shoulders, arms, jaw, thighs, and even feet. When we let go of a physical tension, we also let go of the corresponding negative emotions.

Tension responses are kicked into gear by the sympathetic nervous system, which is in turn activated by the startle reflex. The sympathetic nervous system is the part of our autonomic nervous system that turns on automatically to protect us from perceived danger. In addition to muscular bracing and shallow breathing, other sympathetic nervous system responses include cold hands and feet—due to contraction of the blood vessels—and gastrointestinal discomfort—due to blood shifting away from the digestive centers of the body, which are governed by the parasympathetic system.

The sympathetic nervous system works in concert with the brain's reticular activating system, a part of the body that carries messages from the cerebral cortex—our conscious minds—to our muscles and organs, sounding the alarm. The reticular activating system links the mind—the brain's cortex—and the body into a mutual feedback loop. Its activity accounts for how thoughts produce direct visceral responses in the tissues and vice versa.

The body's endocrine system, regulated by the hypothalamus and the pituitary, also collaborates with the sympathetic nervous system. When the startle reflex sounds the alarm, the hypothalamus initiates endocrine changes that release adrenaline and noradrenaline from the medulla of the adrenal glands, producing the adrenaline rush that characterizes responses to danger and challenge.

WHEN TENSION BECOMES CHRONIC

In the fight-or-flight response, the body and brain systems all focus on a single goal: *action!* If we can act effectively, we can escape or overcome the danger. Once the danger is overcome, the tension in our bodies can release, our circulation can return to normal, our digestive functions can resume, our hormones can rebalance, our anger or fear can dissipate, and we can move toward homeostasis. Tension has served its purpose—of helping us cope—and it can dissipate without self-destructive consequences.

But when we feel that we cannot act and the startle reflex cannot trigger the body-mind into a *temporary* state of alarm that helps us deal with and then resolve the danger at hand, we are relentlessly stressed. We may just end up in a permanent startle reflex if there is no way to get out of daily traffic jams, the treadmill of work, controlling employers and colleagues, nagging family members, or an endless inner dialogue of self-criticism. When it feels as though our life is under the control of forces over which we have no control and the demand for action in response to danger is constant and never-ending, all our systems stay stuck on "on." Our muscles, rather than tightening briefly and then relaxing, stay tight. They develop a *habit of tension.* This causes them to tire more and more easily. We feel this muscle fatigue as pain. If life breeds a habit of tension in us, eventually our body wears down and habitual tension turns into habitual pain.

WHEN CHRONIC TENSION BECOMES UNCONSCIOUS

We are not always conscious of stress and may be in a constant state of stress without realizing it. You may think, "I have chronic pain, but I am not in a constant state of stress. What's more, I don't feel muscle tension, but I *am* in pain! So what's causing it?"

Any condition that becomes continuous also tends to become unconscious. Have you ever entered a quiet room and remarked to yourself that you hadn't realized how noisy things were around you until the moment things became more peaceful? After spending a few days on vacation, have you ever said to yourself that you had no idea how wound up you really were until you took some time to unwind? In these cases, *a condition has become unconscious because you were habituated to it.* That condition becomes conscious only when something causes your situation to change. Similarly, startle-reflex stress can become so endemic that we lose consciousness of it. We no longer think that the level of anxiety or irritability we feel is abnormal. We may even deny to others—and to ourselves—that we feel anxious, fearful, irritable, or angry. Why? Because the way we feel has become the norm. We don't expect things to be different, and so the way we feel is fine. Under these conditions, we notice that we are nervous, anxious, or angry only when we become more than usually nervous, anxious, or angry. We deny the reality of our tension. We have all seen this form of denial in others. Have you ever advised a friend to relax, and he yelled back at you, with evident irritation, "I am relaxed!" By his very action, he has proven that he was not.

All four of the individuals described in chapter 1 registered feelings of reduced pain, along with enhanced calm and peace, when they worked on releasing the physiological stress that had accumulated in their bodies. They discovered that their stress responses were chronic and unconscious. They had not been aware of how tension was creating their pain.

Just as we may no longer consciously feel our emotional and mental tensions, we may also no longer consciously register our body's tension. We may notice it only when our body gets tighter than usual, for example when the straw breaks the camel's back at work and suddenly we have a roaring headache. The unconscious nature of habitual stress is one of the reasons that its effects can be so insidiously destructive. Pain seems to come out of the blue, but in fact the chances are that it has been creeping up on us for a while.

Even when our daily life seems to be running smoothly, we can still suffer from the physical, mental, and emotional ramifications of stress due to an overly active fight-or-flight response. Our bodies and minds are creatures of habit. Once you have a habit of stress, you can find it difficult to let go of it. Let's say you've spent fifteen years in a high-pressure job or raising children. Let's say those stresses are now gone. Your job is pleasant, or you're retired. Your children have left the nest or are no longer as demanding, and you have time on your hands. Even so, you find yourself unable to sleep at night, and you stay up worrying about one thing or another. Let's say you grew up having to perform for your parents, and you learned to put the squeeze on yourself so as to shine for them. Your parents have long ago abandoned their role as authorities in your life, yet you still feel driven to perform, and you can't stop. Why? You have a habit of chronic tension.

This tension is as much physical as it is mental. Your muscles have something called "muscle memory." They have learned, through years of experience, to tense up in preparation for danger, and they no longer know how to let go. This tension is beyond your conscious control, *unless you retrain your muscles*. And so, because your body is chronically tight, your physical tension causes you to feel nervous or irritable and to be mentally hyperactive and vigilant. Melissa's chronic fibromyalgia pain was as much the result of habitual muscular tension over which she had lost control as it was the result of anxiety that triggered her muscles into a contraction response. Habitual physical tension drove her into continual anxiety, which in turn fed her physical tension. She could not get a handle on this vicious cycle until she practiced deep physiological relaxation through breath awareness work.

Our angry or anxious thoughts and feelings are the companions of physical tension. We may feel nervous, anxious, upset, or angry; our mind may race from one thought to another; or we may feel overextended, even when we no longer have strong reasons for feeling and thinking this way—all because our muscles have a bad habit of tension. And so . . . we feel pain.

Because muscle tension can become habitual and chronic, and because it is often a consequence of emotional and mental stress, consciously learning to recognize and reduce physical tension responses can be a highly efficient way of addressing all forms of stress. Even when stress is ultimately caused by emotional reactions to life's events, you may be able to address it through body reeducation rather than emotional counseling. Stress-based emotions always manifest as physiological tensions. Releasing those tensions helps you both to release pain and to deal with the emotional stresses that underlie the pain.

Reducing chronic pain requires that you learn how to take yourself out of the startle reflex. You need to learn how to detach from bodily reactions of tension that are habitually beyond your conscious control but that you can learn to master. In this process, you will learn to address stress where it resides in your body.

How Chronic Tension Creates Pain

Chronically tight muscles are painful. They can also create pain in other parts of the body. Pain is a result of excess internal bodily pressure from muscles that are themselves too tight or that have been excessively strained and stretched by tight muscles that connect to them. A tight muscle in the neck, for example, can cause low back strain. Some pain is also a result of adhesions—areas where layers of body tissue stick together and no longer glide freely—and of strains in the connective tissue web that envelops and supports all the tissues and organs of our body, including muscle tissues. Connective tissue adhesions in the hip can radiate up to the shoulder, restricting motion and predisposing a person to shoulder injuries. Tension in one part of the body creates tension in other parts.

Tense muscles, along with the connective tissue that envelops them, also put pressure on other structures they connect to, envelop, and support. These structures include the nerves, the arteries and veins that feed them, and the bones. Irritation of the nerves and reduced blood supply to muscles create and aggravate pain. Chronically contracted muscles and connective tissue adhesions put pressure on the joints and bones, promoting joint, bone, and disc pain. Joint pain, for example in the hip or the knee, is often the result of imbalances and tensions within the muscles and connective tissue, or fascia, that connect to those joints. Similarly, excessive muscular tension can result in a herniated disc, where two vertebrae are squeezed so much that the gel cushion between them, known as the intervertebral disc, extrudes beyond the vertebrae and impinges on the surrounding nerves. Excess muscle tension and connective tissue stress can also contribute to osteoarthritis, since the calcification typical of osteoarthritis is in part the body's self-protective response to excess pressure put onto the bones.

Even where pain is not a direct result of too great neuromuscular stress, as in rheumatoid arthritis or some forms of osteoarthritis, neuromuscular tension will significantly aggravate those pain syndromes, and releasing tension can reduce pain levels markedly.

Other aspects of stress also contribute to pain. For example, in situations of prolonged stress, the hypothalamus activates the pituitary to release additional hormones, some of which can cause inflammation. An overactive sympathetic nervous system also inhibits the activity of the parasympathetic nervous system, which is responsible for proper digestion. If digestion suffers, the digestive organs can atrophy, making the musculature and connective tissue surrounding these organs more prone to inflammation. Under chronic stress, the reticular activating system continues to send the alarm to muscles and organs, which triggers more fear, anxiety, and worrisome thoughts, resulting in a continuously stressed feedback loop.

WHEN STRESS BEGINS AS PHYSICAL TENSION

Stress and pain can have a purely physiological origin. For example, some people develop chronic pain from poor posture. They sit and stand with their head too far forward of their neck, and eventually this imbalance creates enough pressure on the spine to herniate a disc. In this case, chronic pain seems to start independently of any fight-or-flight response or of the stress with which that response is associated. Yet poor posture, and inefficient movement patterns in general, are stressful to the body: they contribute to major physiological tensions, because the less well-aligned the body is, the more effort and tension it must use to accomplish anything.

Poor posture creates muscle tension. Poor posture is another term for misalignment. We are aligned when our bones do most of their assigned job of supporting our weight. They do this when they stack up balanced one upon the other: the head upon the spine, the spine upon the pelvis, and so on. When they are misaligned, however, they fail to support our weight; then our muscles, which are made primarily to guide us through movement, have to take over the job of support from the bones. For example, if our head is forward of our spine instead of balancing directly over our spine, our muscles have to hold our head up against the pull of gravity. Because muscles aren't meant to perform this function, they work too hard and become tense, or stressed. Muscle tension also activates other elements of the stress response: a sense of physiological, mental, and emotional discomfort, decreased ability to respond creatively to challenges, and decreased ability to focus. The muscle tension that results from poor posture breeds mental and emotional stress, which in turn breeds more physical tension. For example, a person who begins to suffer pain from poor posture also becomes increasingly irritable or anxious as a result. Bodily tension creates mental and emotional tension. This mental and emotional tension—expressed as frustration and anxiety—then creates increased muscle tension and further pain.

Most people are unaware of the profoundly stressful effect of poor posture and inefficient movement. Our culturally accepted notions of stress focus too much on mental and emotional sources of stress and on the objective factors in our situations that trigger these stresses, and overlook the very real importance of the body. The way the body feels affects every part of our lives. Poor posture and inefficient movement are endemic in our society, and the physical, mental, and emotional cost is high.

The more sedentary we are, the more likely we are to suffer from the stress of poor alignment and inefficient movement. We evolved to use our bodies efficiently by using them a great deal and in variable conditions that—unlike modern city streets and ergonomic chairs—demanded body awareness and skill. Today, we hardly use our bodies. Pete Egoscue is an anatomical physiologist whose exercise therapy program for chronic pain has been acclaimed worldwide, and whom famed golf champion Jack Nicklaus credits with totally changing his life. In *The Egoscue Method of Health Through Motion*, Egoscue points out that our culture gives body movement virtually no importance. The result is an epidemic of serious chronic pain disorders that reflect underuse of the body.

Frequent, varied movement is a principal mechanism through which the body learns how to be free of stress by finding alignment. Conscious awareness of the importance of alignment in maintaining health and vitality can also contribute to a healthy body. Yet our culture is so overfocused on consumption, leisure, and mental pursuits that it pays little attention to the importance of learning alignment. In American schools, children slouch any which way over their desks. In contrast, in Europe and the East, children are taught to sit erect in school, and educators there recognize that postural alignment plays an important role in overall mental and emotional focus and clarity. Once we give our bodies greater importance and cultivate stress-free, focused living habits, we reduce the physiological stresses that cause us to underperform and to be unhealthy.

Traumas from injuries and accidents are another form of stress with a physiological origin. Accidents overwhelm the body's ability to respond creatively, and the stresses they cause can become chronic through the body's muscle memory. It is the muscle memory of an accident, rather than the accident itself, that makes healing difficult. Muscles traumatized by a sudden blow are often unable to return to their original position and continue to behave as though the blow were being experienced again and again. In much the same way that a child who was abandoned will later see abandonment in adult situations, so too muscles that have been injured will continue to act traumatized long after the source of trauma is gone. The muscles act as though their reaction pattern had been frozen in time. Like a broken record, they keep on repeating their contraction reaction to a past experience. Traumatic muscle memories make healing difficult and contribute to a chronic stress response within the body, which perceives itself as being in danger long after the danger is past. Releasing tensions associated with old traumas can help heal seemingly intractable problems related to accidents and injuries.

RECOMMENDATIONS

Any technique that reduces one form of stress, and therefore of pain, will tend to reduce the others. We can calm our mental and emotional stress by learning how to manage or change the physical tensions that are their physiological expressions in the body. And we can reduce physiological stress by addressing the thoughts or emotions that are responsible for triggering muscular and connective tissue stress.

But the most efficient route to alleviating the stress that underlies pain, whether that stress is originally of physical or mental and emotional origin, is through the *body* rather than the mind. Body-centered techniques enable you to address stress where it manifests in the body and to reduce or eliminate the chronic pain that results from stress. These techniques have nothing in common with physical exercise, and this book does not provide a guide to rehabilitation through physical exercise. It offers techniques to enhance and improve your physical self-awareness in a way that spontaneously generates a healing response. As you gain physical self-awareness, you will begin to understand and gain control over all sources of stress in your life. Ultimately, the body expresses your mental and emotional lives, and your mental and emotional lives express themselves through your body. Understanding this mind-body connection more clearly, and how it is played out in the dance of stress, is the subject of chapter 3.

FURTHER READING

Ken Pelletier, *Mind as Healer, Mind as Slayer* (New York: Dell, 1977). Written by a professor of medicine, this is an excellent exploration of how mental, emotional, and physical stress affects the body.

Hans Selye, *The Stress of Life* (New York: McGraw-Hill, 1956). The classic on stress by the man who has shaped our modern understanding of what stress is.

3

STRESS: A MIND-BODY DANCE

Because all stresses register themselves as habits of neuromuscular tension, a body-centered strategy for healing from chronic pain will offer you the most direct approach for beginning to understand how to heal. These habits are largely *unconscious*, and working with the body helps you to make them conscious and control them. The body is, in a sense, a series of unconscious habits. The emotional and mental stresses that contribute to pain form part of this substratum of unconscious habits, and they tend to be registered as bodily reactions rather than as conscious feelings and thoughts. The emotions and thoughts that create the most tension in our lives are those we repress. Body-centered techniques can help bring repressed emotions to consciousness, resolve them, and release chronic pain.

One of my clients, Jim, suffered from chronic neck pain but could find no source for it in his life situation. Things at home were harmonious, he said, and though his work was strenuous, he insisted he enjoyed it. Yes, he said, there were problems on the job, but they were most likely his fault, and he could deal with that. Yet when we worked with helping him to develop body awareness and release physical tension, he began to feel emotions hidden beneath the surface, to admit to himself that his work situation was not acceptable. When he decided that he would have to quit his job, his pain began to lessen.

If I had recognized that my client needed to quit his job and had told him this before he came to that recognition on his own, he might well have gone into denial and rejected my advice. He needed to discover his own truth, to bring it to consciousness for himself. He did that by relaxing into his body's sensations. *The body is a reservoir for thoughts and feelings that are not conscious and that may, precisely because they are unconscious, hold the key to resolving physical pain.* By feeling his body more clearly, and releasing tensions in his body, my client brought unconscious emotional issues to the surface. Learning how to feel your body more directly can help you too connect to and resolve emotional and mental stresses of which you may be unaware and that may contribute directly to pain.

THE BODY STORES UNCONSCIOUS FEELINGS

We sometimes recognize that our bodies are telling us something about how we feel emotionally. Physical pain can signal this realization. Turns of phrase such as "He's a pain in the neck" and "She gives me a headache" tell us that we are having an emotional reaction to a person, and that this reaction is causing us physical pain. Generally, we feel this pain because we do not fully express some emotion over which we feel conflict. For example, we hold on tight inside to keep from exploding with irritation or hurt at a family member, perhaps because we are afraid of that person's reaction: criticism, teasing, or even anger or violence. Because these reactions are too frightening to contemplate, we shut up rather than speak up. In our bodies, however, we feel the tension of our failure to speak out. Or perhaps we have a habit of self-criticism and continually minimize our own opinions. Everyone else is right, and we're wrong. So we shut up and berate ourselves, but we burn inside.

Muscular tension can be a defensive way of holding back or controlling thoughts and emotions about which we feel ambivalent. Emotions express themselves by moving through the body—the word "emotion" comes from the Latin word meaning to "move out"—and muscle tension can effectively inhibit emotions from coming to the fore. This is one reason why some chronic pain syndromes seem to carry a marked demographic bias. For example, 80 percent of the people who suffer from TMJ syndrome are women. TMJ—short for temporomandibular joint—syndrome affects the jaw and can cause jaw clicking, pain, malocclusion, headaches, impaired hearing, dizziness, and nausea, among other symptoms. This syndrome usually involves imbalances and tensions in the muscles controlling the jaw, which is also the gateway for verbalization. Women are more susceptible to TMJ syndrome than men because they have greater difficulties than men feeling self-confident and comfortable about their opinions and power, especially in situations that may involve potential conflict with others. They demonstrate their feelings of conflict by restricting their avenue of expression—clamping down in the jaw. In a similar vein, 85 percent of fibromyalgia sufferers are women. Studies indicate that a disproportionately high percentage of these women have suffered childhood physical or sexual abuse. Perhaps they learned through years of fear to contract into themselves to try to avoid feeling the violence they suffered.

If we were taught to shut up rather than speak up as children, or to hold back rather than express, we may have developed a habit of chronic muscular tension that blocks us from free self-expression of any kind. If that chronic tension finds release through bodywork, suppressed emotions may flow up quite spontaneously. Massage therapists, yoga teachers, movement therapists, craniosacral therapists, Reiki practitioners, and other bodyworkers are familiar with this fact. It is not uncommon for clients receiving massage or manual therapy suddenly to burst into tears of anguish or sorrow, or to express violent anger, as the physiological tension of their bodies lets go.

The suppressed emotional pain that underlies and causes physiological tension is best addressed indirectly, through the body. A variety of schools of body-centered therapy for emotional healing have developed. What is suppressed cannot very readily be called up through verbal therapy, but it can be activated and released through neuromuscular release. In psychology, Wilhelm Reich, an associate of Sigmund Freud who lived during the first part of the twentieth century, was the first professional psychologist in the United States to develop a systematic manual approach to releasing muscle tension and promoting emotional healing and empowerment. He pioneered the use of bodywork to help patients let go of confining emotional patterns and release the defensive emotional armor that people put up that is also a tightening of muscle tissue that holds back and deadens feeling.

Alexander Lowen, the founder of bioenergetics and at one point a student of Reich, further developed Reich's insights. He elaborated a brilliant, powerful analysis of personalities in which each personality type was associated with specific areas of the body—the neck, chest, pelvis, and so on—that were rigid with tension. He showed how these frozen areas of neuromuscular rigidity defend a person against feeling core emotions over which that person has conflict while acting as unconscious motivators in behavior. The basic principle of Lowen's work, as of Reich's, was to help a person get in touch with repressed emotions by means of a combination of physical movement and manual pressure on tight tissues, to release the physiological tensions that hold emotions back. According to this approach, emotional empowerment and maturity develop as a result of freeing up suppressed emotions, since this process helps a person develop a less defended, more secure approach to daily living.

Today, many body-centered therapists help clients heal by locating and releasing their neuromuscular tensions. When neuromuscular blocks give way under manual or energetic pressure, clients frequently recall significant charged experiences that were buried in their unconscious. Afterward, people usually feel physically lighter, emotionally unburdened, and more mentally centered.

Reich's and Lowen's work focused on emotional rather than physical healing, but their body-centered approach reminds us that body tensions that create pain can express unresolved emotional issues and that these emotions will in some instances let go simultaneously with physiological release. The body itself does not seem to be more physical than mental and emotional, nor more mental and emotional than physical. The body is a somatic reservoir of thoughts, feelings, and images. Not only are emotions physical sensations, they can be identical to tension or blockage in the tissues!

MIND AND BODY ARE ONE:
THE SCIENTIFIC EVIDENCE

The body is a source of thoughts and feelings, and the mind is not separate from the body. This truth is so fundamental, and so contrary to our cultural assumptions, that fully understanding it radically changes the way we approach healing from chronic pain. We need to grant the body its full status as a source of intelligence, guidance, and wisdom in our lives, and as a powerful ally in creating change, growth, and healing. Mind is body, and body is mind.

Our everyday language tells us that mind and body are intermingled. "She died of a broken heart"; "He makes me throw up"; "My boss gives me an ulcer." Such expressions acknowledge that our thoughts, emotions, and physical states blend together. Throughout history, many traditions have echoed this wisdom of common sense recorded in language. Oriental medicine finds a connection between physiological and emotional imbalances, and acupuncture theory sees an intimate link between emotional patterns and meridian imbalances. Similarly, native traditions have for centuries felt that spiritual and physical healing were one. Yet despite these traditions, our cultural view of the mind-body connection is strongly influenced by the orientation of seventeenth-century French philosopher René Descartes, who first articulated that mind and body were separate and that the mind was superior to the body. Modern science traces its origins to Descartes, and to the idea that mind and matter belong to different realms. The mind thinks, but the body follows the laws of the material realm. Being material, it doesn't think. It's just a thing.

This bifurcation of a human being into different mental and material aspects has resulted in a peculiar schizophrenia in our thinking. We alternate uneasily between two views, sometimes seeing our mental processes as totally divorced from our body and other times reducing all mental events to processes of a dumb, unthinking, and purely material, mechanical realm. When we adopt the first approach, our thoughts and feelings seem to be uniquely mental phenomena, and we discount the strong synergistic influence that our thoughts and viscera have on each other. We refuse to see that our minds have a strong influence on our bodies. We view the body as a machine and reject the idea that it can affect our thoughts. Since materialism has become the dominant force in our technologically oriented age, however, we more frequently take the second approach and reduce the mind to a purely physical or mechanical phenomenon governed by the laws of matter, our biochemistry, and electrical wiring. In this way, our minds, just like the rest of us, become part of the material world. We tell ourselves we are depressed, anxious, or nervous because our biochemistry or electrical wiring is malfunctioning, as if we had no control over our minds. We identify the mind with a very specific part of the body—namely, the brain—which operates like the rest of the body, as part of the material domain, as if it were some fancy piece of machinery under external causal law.

Whether we see the mind as something that is separate from and irreducible to a purely physical state, or whether we see it as being identical with a purely material brain, we assume that anything that happens to our bodies, including physical pain, is purely physical and should therefore be susceptible to a purely physical solution: injecting chemicals or undergoing surgery, for instance. But this attitude not only defies everyday experience, it has also been scientifically proven to be completely invalid.

Science unequivocally proves *both* that mind and body are completely intertwined *and* that the body is not a thing but rather a working intelligence. So we have to recognize that *the body is not purely physical* and that *the mind is neither purely mental nor a physical reality that is confined to the brain*. Rather, *the mind is in the body, and the body is embodied mind*. The body is a powerful vehicle for self-knowledge, self-transformation, and self-healing, on physical, mental, emotional, and spiritual levels.

The clearest demonstration of the fact that body is mind and mind is somatic comes through the work of scientific researcher Dr. Candace Pert, extensively described in her book *Molecules of Emotion*. Dr. Pert has made a lifelong study of the chemical links between physical structures and emotional experiences. She was responsible for initiating research that uncovered the chemical processes that trigger our moods and experiences. In the early 1970s, Pert's work as an undergraduate researcher focused on finding the receptor—a structure on the surface of the cell—that opiate drugs such as morphine and opium bond to when they enter the body and that triggers a mood-altering response in the body. Biochemicals that influence the body do so by attaching to specific receptors on the cell, which in turn stimulate a series of cellular reactions. In line with leading scientific assumptions that emotions are mental phenomena restricted to the brain, Dr. Pert hypothesized that the substances to which these bliss-triggering drugs linked would be found primarily or solely within the limbic part of the brain that scientific orthodoxy says governs our emotions. She discovered, however, that this was not the case and that those substances are in *every* part of the body. The implication was that the emotion, in this case bliss, is neither generated by nor limited to the brain. Rather, it is generated by and resides in cells throughout the body. In other words, *it is the body, not just the brain, that feels emotions.*

Dr. Pert's findings resulted in further research that led to the discovery in 1976 of endorphins, natural opiates within the body that internally generate feelings of well-being and bliss. These endorphins, along with their receptor sites on cells, exist not only within the emotional centers of the brain but throughout the entire body.

Endorphins are one of a class of peptides, informational substances that bind to a receptor, acting as stimuli that trigger a chain of responses. Neuropeptides are stimuli associated with the specific biochemical responses that trigger various states of mind. Dr. Pert's research led to the discovery that neuropeptides—what might be called the molecules of emotion or the biochemical substrate of emotion—exist not only in the brain but also in the blood, organs, bones, and muscles. The conclusion is inevitable: all our cells are intelligent entities, and our emotions spread themselves throughout our bodies. The idea that our mind is *in* our brain is an outmoded idea peculiar to Western tradition. The mind is not a function of the brain but a flow of information passing through the body that takes place mostly out of our conscious awareness. The subconscious mind is actually the body itself.

Emotions and thoughts come from the body as much as they do from the brain. The body thinks and feels! This scientific finding, which you will find repeatedly corroborated by anecdotal evidence from clients in following chapters and which developed as a result of Dr. Pert's research, has also been dramatically demonstrated in the experiences of recipients of organ transplants. Some of these recipients report having experiences, feelings, and thoughts that are foreign to them but that belonged to the organ donors. For example, one vegetarian organ recipient dreams of eating hamburgers, which the donor ate regularly! Apparently such thoughts are being transmitted through the donor organ to the minds of the recipients.

Given Dr. Pert's research—and the evidence that the body is itself a field of thoughts and emotions—it seems logical to assume that bodywork could elicit emotions and thoughts lodged within the subconscious mind of the body. What's more, Dr. Pert's research encourages us to view the body as a somatic reservoir of unconscious thoughts and feelings, and to consider the possibility that sometimes the body's behavior, including its pain syndromes, is a symbolic statement of unconscious thoughts and emotions that can be perceived through the body. As we shall see in later chapters, it is sometimes possible to talk to the body's tissues and, through this process, to generate healing responses.

RECOMMENDATIONS

Developing heightened body awareness is the royal road to reducing chronic pain. The body is the point of intersection for all the forces in our lives that create physical pain. The body reflects the interactions of all the stresses in our lives and is also the seat of unconscious processes that contribute to pain. By being more present to the body, we make the unconscious conscious and eventually regain control over the body.

Making the unconscious conscious begins on the simplest level, with becoming conscious of physical habits that create tension and pain. These habits are the subject of Part II of this book, chapters 4 through 9, which looks directly at *how to release physical tension patterns that create neuromuscular stress*. Chapters 4 and 5 look at habits of breathing, how they create tension, and how to change them so as to foster deepened muscle relaxation. Improving breathing patterns can have a dramatic and long-lasting impact on pain reduction. Chapters 6 and 7 explore how misalignment can create excess neuromuscular tension and stress, and how to improve alignment. This process also reduces muscle tension and therefore pain. Chapters 8 and 9 explore how we sometimes work too hard with our bodies and how learning to reduce the overall effort our muscles exert in making movements reduces neuromuscular tension. This results not only in major pain reduction, but also in feelings of increased fluidity and grace and a sense of emotional peace and security.

Any reduction in neuromuscular tension will have a significant positive effect on emotional and mental functioning. Reducing physiological tension enables you to manage mental and emotional stress more effectively, which reduces the incidence of stress and therefore pain. Chapters 4 through 9 explain the emotional and mental changes that accompany learning how to reduce and release physiological tensions.

Part III of this book, chapters 10 through 15, explores more directly the *emotional and mental dimensions of stress reduction that are raised through enhanced body awareness*. The muscles can store unconscious feelings, and the body is part of our intelligence. Heightening body awareness through reducing physiological tensions may sometimes result in insights about feelings that can reduce chronic pain. Chapters 10 through 12 explore the fascinating process by which unconscious emotional material is suppressed through physiological tension and released through body self-awareness.

Specific, culturally endorsed thought patterns and emotional attitudes can create chronic stress and contribute to pain. Our attempt to adhere to attitudes with which we are in conflict creates pain. Becoming aware of the conflict between cultural rules and our own needs helps resolve this conflict and is the focus of chapters 13 through 15.

Part II begins with a strictly physical approach to tension reduction that also leads you naturally and organically into beginning to become conscious of the emotional content of your body, which is the subject of Part III. Becoming more present to your body makes you more present to how you feel and therefore to emotional and mental issues that may be contributing to neuromuscular stress. The more familiar you become with your body, the more obvious it becomes that it is through the body that you feel and register your mental and emotional reactions to life. Through using the body to get more thoroughly in touch with these reactions, you promote further physical healing. You'll progress in this book from learning about purely physiological tension reduction in chapters 4 through 9, to feeling emotions in the body in chapters 10 through 12, to exploring how thoughts and emotions can actually create bodily pain or freedom from pain in chapters 13 through 15.

In the following chapters you will find a great many techniques for self-healing from chronic pain. Every technique presented here can provide some help in reducing chronic pain. At the same time, each individual is unique, and in each individual case of chronic pain, there are both primary and secondary factors that contribute to that pain. For some people, the breathing techniques in chapters 4 and 5 will open a doorway to major relief. For others, it may be reducing tension through alignment training presented in chapters 6 and 7, or through muscle release techniques presented in chapters 8 and 9, that is critical. For yet others, emotional release or insight may provide the fundamental key. The chapters are organized so that each can be read separately, and you may be drawn to one section more than another. Nonetheless, I advise you to begin by reading and using each chapter in succession. The art of working with your body to reduce pain is just that: an art. To develop it fully, begin by reading and using each chapter in succession. Then go back and work with the chapters that seem to provide the most important keys to your own self-healing. You are likely to find that the key that seems most important at one time will recede into the background at another, to be superseded by yet another approach that may have held little appeal for you initially.

Keep in mind that healing is a process. It involves changing the patterns of a lifetime. Once you feel the effect of the self-healing tools provided in each chapter, you will want to make them a regular part of your life: today, tomorrow, next month, next year, and ten years from now. Your commitment to the process will not only bring you back to full health, it will also improve your health beyond what you had thought possible. If you are particularly drawn to certain techniques I advocate, you may want to explore that technique in further depth; each chapter also includes references that allow you to do that.

And now, on to the first key to healing from chronic pain: breathing.

FURTHER READING

Alexander Lowen, *The Language of the Body* (New York: Collier Macmillan, 1958). A fascinating account, by the creator of Bioenergetics, of the relationship between patterns of neuromuscular stress and personality dynamics.

Candace Pert, *Molecules of Emotion: The Science Behind Mind-Body Medicine* (New York: Simon & Schuster, 1999). The author's personal story of her experiences researching, discovering, and disseminating information on the link between neuropeptides and emotions.

Wilhelm Reich, *Character Analysis* (New York: Orgone Institute Press, 1949). A classic by the founder of modern body-centered therapy.

Part II

YOUR
BODY

LETTING GO
OF PHYSICAL STRESS

4

HOW YOUR BODY BREATHES

The way you breathe is probably the single most important factor influencing your health. Because how you breathe is intimately related to the tension in your body, and because it affects your functioning at deep organic levels, breathing patterns have a profound effect on how easily you move, whether you feel pain, and how much pain you feel. Less than 10 percent of the population breathes efficiently. Yet by learning to breathe more efficiently and easily, you can easily reduce your level of pain, increase your ease of movement and sense of well-being, develop greater emotional calm, and vastly improve your general health.

The breath can be smooth or jerky, soft or harsh, deep or shallow, free or restricted. If your breathing is restricted—if it is shallow and fast rather than deep and slow, if it is uneven or labored, and if you have a tendency to hold your breath—then you are suffering from the long-term consequences of stress. Restricted, shallow breathing is triggered by the fight-or-flight response. When it becomes chronic, the restriction in your breath translates directly into increased effort, anxiety or frustration, decreased mobility, and increased pain.

Right now, you can discover for yourself how restricted breathing increases tension. Here is a simple experiment. Start by sitting in a chair. Stand up several times. The first time you stand up, consciously hold your breath while you do so. Do this now. The second time you stand up, breathe in by taking a nice deep inhalation as you stand up, at the very moment that you move from sitting to standing. Repeat this experiment several times, alternating between holding your breath as you stand up and taking a full inhalation as you stand. Do you notice a difference between the two? If you breathe in as you stand up, you feel more comfortable and move more easily than if you hold your breath. The reason is that when you breathe, your diaphragm muscle moves properly. When you hold your breath, your diaphragm muscle tenses. You feel this as an increase of effort in your body. Unfortunately, many people hold their breath as they go from sitting to standing. Chances are, they hold their breath in other movements as well. This holding creates stress and contributes to pain.

Let's explore the difference between full, free breathing and restricted breathing as we examine the physiology of proper breathing.

THE PHYSIOLOGY OF BREATHING

When we breathe into our lungs, the respiratory muscles actually draw oxygen into the body. The most important of these muscles is the diaphragm, which is responsible for 75 percent of the respiratory work and so is called a *primary* muscle of respiration. Efficient breathing is called diaphragmatic breathing.

When the diaphragm muscle does its proper share of the work, we breathe well, and our breathing is relaxed and deep. When that muscle does *not* work the way it should, our breathing becomes restricted and labored, and we feel all the consequences of the stress response: physical tension, negative emotions, mental stress, and pain. If you wish to reduce your chronic pain, then make daily, habitual diaphragmatic breathing your goal. You will feel much, much better.

One of the strongest muscles in the body, the double-domed diaphragm sits in the chest like a parachute. It is attached in front to the little bone at the end of the breastbone called the xiphoid process; on the sides, to the cartilage of the seventh through twelfth ribs; and down the front of the spine, to the first, second, third, and fourth lumbar vertebrae. The diaphragm sits below the lungs and the heart and above all the organs of digestion, including the stomach, liver, and gall bladder, pancreas, small intestine, and large intestine. It is connected to all of these organs by connective tissue, a fibrous web that spreads throughout the body and provides structural support for all the organs and muscles.

To get a sense of where your own diaphragm is, place your hands facing each other with fingertips touching, palms down, and with the inside of your hands (your thumbs and index fingers) contacting your sternum. Your hands should be horizontal. The resting position of the diaphragm is just below your hands.

When the diaphragm functions as it is meant to, it moves from this resting position and contracts downward to bring air into the lungs. Then it relaxes, moving back up to its original position as air is expelled from the lungs. When the diaphragm descends and reascends freely, it brings an abundance of vital oxygen into the lungs. The lungs and heart in turn cooperate in transporting this oxygen to the tissues. The deeper our breathing—or the more diaphragmatically we breathe—the more oxygen we take in. This translates into greater oxygenation of the muscles, a vital ingredient in maintaining pain-free tissues. It also results in less stress on the heart—the organ responsible for getting oxygenated blood to the tissues—and a greater flow of vital nutrients to organs, all of which in turn promotes overall tissue health and freedom from pain. When the diaphragm descends fully, it massages and stimulates all the digestive organs that lie below it, squeezing and releasing them like sponges. Diaphragmatic breathing is essential for complete digestion and elimination, as well as for the processing of toxins.

Because poor breathing results in inefficient digestion and assimilation, as well as in a reduced flow of blood and nutrients, it can cause organs to deteriorate. This deterioration communicates itself directly to organ-related muscles and connective tissue, causing nerve, muscle, and connective tissue inflammation, which translates into pain. The potential negative impact of poor breathing is extensive.

How the Diaphragm Affects Other Muscles

Restricted diaphragmatic movement has other effects on major muscle groups throughout the body. Because the diaphragm is such a large, powerful muscle, and because it is intimately related through a web of connective tissue to all the other muscles of the body, *any restriction of the diaphragm's movement translates into muscle tension and connective tissue stress throughout the body*. That means increased effort, discomfort, emotional tension, and eventually pain.

You can see how deeply interconnected and interdependent our muscles are by performing the following experiment. First, stand up. Now tighten your abdominal muscles. Can you feel tension coming into other muscles? Where do you feel the tension? Do you notice changes in your neck, shoulders, back, or legs? Notice what happens to your breathing as well. Now relax your abdomen and tighten your buttocks. Where do you feel the tension? In your back? Thighs? Abdomen? Chest? Now tighten the muscles of your neck and notice what other muscles get tight. Finally, hold your breath and notice how, by stopping breathing and restricting the natural movement of the diaphragm, you tighten muscles throughout your body.

What have you learned? *That tension in any major muscle group in your body creates tension in other muscles.* This is especially true of the diaphragm. When the diaphragm is tight and moves only with effort—when your breathing is not full and deep—other muscles in your body will also be tight. For example, rigidity of the diaphragm can result in tension in the pelvic muscles, which can in turn cause low back and hip pain. Similarly, because the knees depend on the flexibility of the hips and low back, restricted breathing can result in knee pain, including deterioration of cartilage and arthritic deposits. Problems that seem very far removed from the diaphragm can have their origin in diaphragmatic tension. For the same reason, when the diaphragm is relaxed and moves easily, problems with muscles and joints that seem far removed from the diaphragm may be eased.

When the diaphragm muscle is relaxed, it moves easily up and down and the breath is even, steady, deep, soft, and slow. Because the diaphragm moves easily, other muscles in the body are also more likely to move easily. Therefore, *when the breath is soft, deep, and slow, muscles will also tend to be relaxed and movement will be easier.* But when the diaphragm is *not* relaxed, when it moves less freely, the breath becomes uneven, shallow, faster, and more labored. If the diaphragm is tight, other muscles tighten, movement becomes more difficult, and pain becomes more pronounced. Since full, deep, and easy breathing translates into freedom from tension, and tension means pain, what better reason to breathe diaphragmatically than to free yourself of tension and pain! Breathing diaphragmatically—slowly, softly, and deeply—reduces muscle tension throughout the body.

WHEN SECONDARY MUSCLES DO THE WORK MEANT FOR THE DIAPHRAGM

When our bodies are under stress, we tend not to breathe diaphragmatically. When we do not breathe diaphragmatically and the tension of the diaphragm communicates itself through a web of connective tissue to other muscles, which also become tight, the resulting muscle stress creates discomfort and further problems arise because secondary respiratory muscles take over the job of trying to bring oxygen into the body. These muscles of the upper torso, including the chest, neck, and jaw, are not built to do the work of the diaphragm, and they tire easily, which creates upper back, shoulder, neck, and jaw tension and pain, as well as headaches.

People who rely primarily on their secondary respiratory muscles to breathe, rather than on the primary muscle of the diaphragm, are thoracic breathers, or *chest breathers.* Their chests move up and down as they breathe, while the abdomen stays uninvolved. People who suffer from chronic pain, including neck and shoulder pain, are frequently chest breathers.

People who breathe diaphragmatically are *belly breathers.* Their bellies move in and out with the breath while their chests stay relatively quiet. Statistically, diaphragmatic or belly breathers are far less likely than chest breathers to suffer chronic pain.

Because stress almost invariably reflects itself in shallow breathing, the clearest indicator of stress is the habit of chest breathing. By working to shift from chest breathing toward diaphragmatic breathing, you can reverse the sympathetic nervous system's tendency toward hyperarousal. This will go a long way toward reducing the muscular tension and connective tissue stress that underlie most cases of chronic pain. It will also give you a vehicle for feeling more centered and balanced in your life, and less subject to the daily pressures that surround you.

Enhanced mental and emotional calm can reduce stress and therefore physical pain. *Breathing diaphragmatically increases mental focus and emotional calm and decreases physical tension.*

Nowhere is the connection between our physiology and our mental and emotional life more evident than in breathing, which influences our sense of well-being so immensely that numerous spiritual traditions make the breath the golden beacon that guides us to full physical vitality and personal power.

THE LINK BETWEEN YOUR BREATH AND YOUR MIND

The power of the breath for transforming every aspect of our lives has earned it a prominent place both in spiritual traditions and in common parlance. In the biblical tradition, God "breathed" into Adam; the word "spirit" has the same root as the word "respiration"; and the word to "inspire" literally means "to breathe into." In everyday language we acknowledge the importance of the breath when we say that a view is "simply breathtaking," that we "need room to breathe," that someone "takes our breath away," or that at last we can "breathe freely." Every aspect of our lives is reflected in and responds to the quality of our breathing.

Among ancient spiritual traditions, Buddhism and Yoga give a central role to the breath. Each of these disciplines sees its philosophy as simultaneously a science of health, a psychology of mind, a process for maximizing all human capacities, and a vehicle for spiritual growth. Each also feels it has identified *a single* path, through the body, that will simultaneously optimize the functioning of mind, emotions, and body, generate peak performance, and lead to spiritual self-realization. Yoga and Buddhism are profoundly physical and use the physical body as an instrument of self-knowledge through the practices of physical self-awareness and self-mastery based on full, deep, effortless breathing.

When we breathe easily, we feel physically relaxed, emotionally peaceful, mentally focused, and calm. When our breathing is restricted, we feel physically tense, emotionally irritable, fearful, anxious or angry, and mentally hyperactive (our mind chatters nonstop) or confused. As Yoga and Buddhism recognize, there is a *one-to-one correlation among our physical, emotional,* and *mental states.* This correlation can be diagrammed as follows:

**Relaxed breathing = Muscle relaxation =
Peaceful emotions = Mental focus**

and

**Restricted breathing = Muscle Tension =
Negative emotions (fear, anger, etc.) = Mental agitation**

In principle, changing any one of the four variables automatically changes all the others. Each variable entrains the other three.

We have already explored one aspect of this four-way correlation: the connection between breathing patterns and the muscles. As the diagram above indicates, when the breath is relaxed and deep, muscles will be relaxed, and when the breath is restricted, muscles will be tense. Expanding on the four-way correlation defined above, relaxed breathing and muscle relaxation will bring in their train peaceful emotions and mental focus. Restricted breathing and muscle tension will bring in their train negative emotions and mental agitation.

This four-way correlation can be activated by starting with *any one* of the four variables in the equation above. For example, let's say we become emotionally upset—irritated or fearful. This unpleasant emotion automatically translates into physical tension. Our breath becomes shallow and tight, our jaw or chest tightens, our shoulders hunch, or our gut clenches. At the same time, we tend to lose mental focus—our mind starts to race, we get distracted or confused, or we go into a fog. Our emotions trigger a chain reaction in our bodies and our minds. Everyone has had this experience.

Let's say you get caught in a traffic jam and you're late for an important meeting. It's upsetting! While you wait for the car in front of you to budge, you find yourself gripping the wheel with your hands or holding your breath and grinding your teeth: all signs of physical tension. At the same time, you have a hard time concentrating. You flip distractedly from one radio station to another or yell at the person in the passenger seat, telling him or her you can't focus on what he or she is saying, you're too concerned about the traffic! You are mentally as well as physically agitated, and this agitation was triggered by an emotional upset.

Now envisage a different situation, where the chain reaction starts with a loss of mental focus instead of an emotional upset. Suppose you start to obsess mentally over something: how to meet a deadline, how to hit that next golf ball after you messed up on the last two drives, or how to convince a family member of your point of view in a major disagreement. As soon as you start overthinking, other things happen as well. Your muscles tighten up. Perhaps this gives you a headache. Your breath gets shallower. And you become more irritable or anxious. A change in your mental state has triggered changes in your breathing, your muscles, and your emotions.

Each of the four variables—the breath, the muscles, the emotions, and the mental state—has a domino effect on the others. Once one variable changes, they all do. This gives us important information about how better to manage our lives and our health. If we can readily influence one of these variables, we can influence all of them. As it turns out, it is much harder to influence our emotional and mental states directly than it is to influence our muscles and our breathing. Have you ever noticed how difficult it is to talk yourself out of anxiety or anger? Usually you just have to get away from the situation and give yourself time to cool down. When you're obsessing about some-

thing late at night, it is hard to stop, even though you know that obsessing isn't accomplishing anything and you are losing sleep. We
have remarkably little direct control over our thoughts and feelings,
which seem to have a will of their own. But we *can* influence our
breath and our muscles relatively easily. And through doing this we
can *directly* manage how we feel physically and also *indirectly* manage our emotions and our mental states. This is why breath awareness
and breath control can have a profoundly beneficial impact on all levels of stress. When we use breathing to reduce emotional and mental
as well as physical stress, we improve our quality of life, and the improvement will in turn reduce the tensions that result in pain.

Because control of the breath is an efficient tool for mastering our
bodies, minds, and emotions, accelerated learning programs such as
those developed in the 1960s by Bulgarian scientist Georgi Lozanov
use relaxed deep breathing as a foundation for efficient learning.
They are based on the fact that if you can deepen the breath and relax
the body, your mental acuity will improve fourfold. Similarly, according to Charles Garfield, author of *Peak Performance*, top-level athletes
may spend far more time in deep relaxation training than in body
building and practicing their sport. When the Soviets swept the
Olympics in 1970, researchers discovered that it was not steroids that
had made them superior to American athletes, but mental exercises.
American athletes focused 100 percent of their training on physical
activity and competition, while the Soviets spent only about 25 percent in comparable activities and the remaining 75 percent practicing
deep relaxation, including diaphragmatic breathing. The physiological relaxation optimized their mental focus and emotional function
and fine-tuned their bodies' responsiveness.

BREATHING, PHYSICAL HEALING, AND
PERSONAL GROWTH

In the next chapter, you will learn diaphragmatic breathing. Working with breathing involves something more, however, than committing yourself to spending ten or fifteen minutes a day practicing

specific breathing exercises. The key is to *integrate* the diaphragmatic breathing you learn through breathing exercises into how you breathe *throughout* the day.

Breath work is exciting—physically pleasurable, relaxing, and personally enriching. It helps us to change for the better on many levels, all of which in turn enhance physical functioning. I am always astonished at the depth and variety of experiences that clients discover through simple instruction in breathing techniques, as the following story shows.

A few years ago, I was giving a course on chronic pain management for a class of twenty people. It was the first meeting of the course, and I was introducing the participants to some breath awareness exercises for physiological relaxation. The class members were lying on mats on the floor, listening to my voice as I took them through a fifteen-minute meditative exercise whose goal was to deepen and relax the breath. When I asked for feedback at the end of the class, all said that they felt more peaceful and relaxed. Two participants were also surprised at physical changes that had already occurred. One, a sixty-year-old gentleman with unremitting leg pain, said his pain had disappeared for the first time in months while he was following the breathing instructions. The other, a man in his forties, said that while his back usually bothered him whenever he got up from a reclining position, when he stood up after the exercise, he was free of pain.

We continued the breathing work, this time sitting rather than lying down. A woman in her forties, who had great trouble with sitting due to two herniated discs, remarked that her pain lessened markedly. We had spent only half an hour working with the breath, and already we were getting results!

After fielding some more feedback, I sent the class participants home with instructions to do two things. First, every day they were to practice the meditative breathing exercise I had just introduced. Second, they were to become aware of their breathing patterns throughout the day and notice if they breathed shallowly or held their breath. When they noticed that their breathing was restricted, they were to try to breathe more diaphragmatically. I told them that we would share the results of our experiences the next week.

At our next meeting, Jacqueline was the first to speak. Jacqueline suffered from arthritis in the neck and shoulders. She said that she found the meditative breathing extremely relaxing, that it reduced her pain, and that it helped her sleep at night. Jacqueline also remarked that when she remembered to be more aware of her breathing during the day and to breathe more diaphragmatically, it seemed to reduce her pain. Most of the other students said the breath work also helped them relax, manage their pain better, and sometimes significantly reduce their pain.

Donald, a forty-five-year old gentleman with low back pain, also remarked that the breathing helped him manage his emotional reactions. He was an avid baseball fan and often became agitated while watching baseball games on television. This was not only emotionally draining and uncomfortable; it also aggravated his pain. As a result, he had decided during the previous week to practice breathing diaphragmatically while he was watching television. He discovered that by being aware of and managing his breathing, he could enjoy the games fully and yet feel detached enough that he did not become overly excited. As a result, his pain receded.

Marie voiced a similar feeling. Once she had gotten used to breathing diaphragmatically, she had practiced paying attention to her breathing throughout the day, which had resulted in some important realizations. She had discovered an unconscious habit that had been with her for years. When her husband became temperamental and critical with her, she tended to hold her breath or to breathe more quickly and shallowly. No wonder her back bothered her after these arguments!

Marie had decided to focus on relaxing into her breathing when her husband became argumentative. This was not always easy, since her spontaneous reaction was to get tense and anxious. But she kept at it, working on calming herself through breathing regularly and deeply. This helped her to feel more centered, which in turn reduced her back pain. The calmer she became, the less she reacted to her husband's comments and the less defensive she became. Her husband, in turn, seemed to respond to her change in behavior by becoming less critical of her. Their mood at home began to shift, and Marie felt more at peace. By changing her own breathing pattern, Marie not only influenced her own physiology and reduced her pain but changed her environment, which further reduced the tension and stress in her life and also reduced her physical pain.

Another woman commented that observing her breath and working on breathing diaphragmatically whenever she felt her breath getting shallow had made her aware of fears that were driving her behavior. She had begun to realize that tension in her own body triggered the need to reach for another cup of coffee or a cigarette or to yell at one of her children. She noticed that when she could take time to breathe before having that cigarette or when she felt like reacting to her kids, her breath awareness helped her to feel less agitated and more in control, and her pain dissipated.

Finally, one woman expressed a spiritual realization, saying the breath work made her feel more open and grateful toward life. She could just breathe. She didn't have to have all the answers. Focusing on breathing seemed to make her more appreciative, calmer, and physically more comfortable. She was surprised that something as simple as changing her breathing pattern could give rise to such a deep spiritual and emotional change.

Each of these class participants reduced his or her physical pain through breath awareness. In the process each of them also made discoveries that helped minimize overall stress, which in turn further reduced the tension that caused pain.

In some cases, the discoveries people make through breath awareness affect just one dimension of their awareness. They learn to relax more physically, to sleep better, or to be emotionally calmer, but often enough, a person practicing breath awareness uses this practice to heal on multiple layers simultaneously. When Melissa, the fibromyalgia client described in chapter 1, learned how to shift into deeper, slower breathing, she also realized that her constricted breathing was part of a punitive habit of pushing herself out of an unconscious need to perform. Practicing deep, easy breathing helped her see that she could perform better with less tension. It taught her how, by relaxing into her body, she could be more self-nurturing and let go of the thoughts and feelings that drove her to overperform.

In my own case, I quickly noticed that focusing on breathing deeply helped reduce my low back pain. I also began to observe other results. For example, I became aware that I frequently breathed shallowly when engaged in conversation with superiors in the office, or even with family members with whom I was having difficulty communicating. My breath awareness practice made me more aware of my body as a whole, and I also noticed that in these same situations my neck and shoulders tended to get tight and my abdomen to knot up. The tensions were all about one thing: stress when I felt controlled or underappreciated, both in the office and on the home front.

I worked on reducing my physical stress reactions through breath awareness. That helped me to feel calmer and more confident, and my back and neck pain receded. Becoming aware of subliminal body tensions through practicing relaxed breathing also made me aware that I needed to deal with some emotional issues of which I had not been conscious. Even though most people viewed me as independent, resourceful, and self-assertive, I began to realize that inside, I was somewhat fearful of stating my own opinions and needs and of establishing boundaries that worked for me. Once I became clearer about these issues, I could work on addressing them directly. When I noticed myself getting tense, I made a point of asking myself whether I was respecting my own boundaries. Doing this gradually reduced the stress of my life and played an important role in further reducing my pain. All of these insights were triggered by breath awareness work.

RECOMMENDATIONS

When I teach breath awareness, I ask people to follow a fourfold process. First, they observe their own breathing, answering for themselves a series of questions I give them about their breathing patterns. By doing this, they find out things about themselves that they had never known: how deeply or shallowly they breathe, how often they hold their breath, and what events, thoughts, and emotions trigger changes in their breathing patterns.

Second, I ask students to practice every day a specific fifteen-to-twenty-minute meditative breathing exercise that gives them the experience of what relaxed, diaphragmatic breathing feels like and begins to change some of their unconscious, stressful breathing habits.

Third, students begin to integrate the meditative breathing that they have learned into simple daily activities. They practice breathing more easily and deeply while walking the dog, washing dishes, and watching television. Eventually, they learn through this practice how to breathe more calmly and deeply while in the midst of their daily routine.

Fourth, they observe the effect that this change in breathing habits has on various aspects of their lives: their level of pain, their sense of emotional or mental peace, their ability to deal with stress. The more they follow this process, the more they commit to developing an ongoing habit of breath awareness and diaphragmatic breathing and to integrating this practice into every aspect of their lives.

As you work with your breathing, you will follow the same process. The next chapter will guide you along this path.

FURTHER READING

Ingrid Bacci, *The Art of Effortless Living* (New York: Perigee, 2002). This book by the author provides extensive and inspiring anecdotal evidence of the power of breath awareness for reducing stress.

Donna Farhi, *The Breathing Book* (New York: Henry Holt, 1996). An in-depth exploration of both the physiology of breathing and techniques for opening up the breath.

5

BREATHING YOUR WAY TO EASE

Take the time to make a thorough initial evaluation of your breathing habits by completing the simple self-test below. Analyzing your own breathing patterns establishes a starting point that will help you to recognize how the way you breathe may be creating pain, and how quickly you improve as you work with breath awareness training.

HOW DO YOU BREATHE?

1. Count your breaths for a full minute. As you do this, try not to change the way you breathe. You are interested in finding out about yourself, not in doing things the "right" way. Put down this book now and count your breaths for one minute exactly, keeping time with a second hand on a watch or clock. Remember to breathe exactly as you do normally, without altering your breathing to try to breathe in a way that you might feel is more correct. Then make a record of how many breaths you breathed.

How many breaths did you take? Most people breathe somewhere between 11 and 30 breaths a minute. When your body breathes in a fully relaxed manner, however—when it breathes deeply and easily—you will tend to breathe between 4 and 10 breaths a minute. If you do not breathe this slowly, and very few people do, do not be alarmed.

You have simply discovered that your breathing habits are probably contributing to your pain. With this new knowledge, you can develop breathing habits that will reduce your pain and improve the way you feel.

2. *Notice if you breathe into your chest or your belly.* Put one hand on your chest and one hand over your belly. Breathe normally and take a few minutes to answer each of the following questions. Be sure to take all the time you need to answer these questions to your full satisfaction:

a. Does your *chest* rise with the in breath and fall with the out breath?
b. Does your *belly* rise with the in breath and fall with the out breath?
c. Does your chest rise more than your belly, or does your belly rise more than your chest?
d. Do both your chest and belly rise, or does only your chest rise, or only your belly?
e. Does something different from the above happen? For example, does your belly expand with the out breath and contract with the in breath?

If you are a "chest breather," your chest will move more than your belly as you breathe in. If you are a "belly breather," your belly will move more as you breathe in. Are you a chest breather or a belly breather? Belly breathers tend to breathe more diaphragmatically than chest breathers. Once you have learned to breathe fully and easily, your chest will move only slightly, and your belly will move more, going out with the in breath and in with the out breath.

3. *Ask yourself if you ever hold your breath.* If so, do you do this frequently, sometimes, or almost never? Many people hold their breath frequently and unconsciously, not only under situations of extreme stress but even in simple activities: as they get up out of a chair or pick up a box, or while engaged in a conversation with someone they want to impress or with whom they disagree. Notice how you

breathe in these types of circumstances, as well as in other routine activities.

4. *Ask yourself if you ever feel short of breath.* Do you feel this way frequently, sometimes, or almost never? The more frequently you feel out of breath, the more likely your breathing is restricted.

5. *Notice whether your breath is calm, regular and even, or a little ragged and punctuated by stops and starts.* Full diaphragmatic breathing is even, regular, and calm, while restricted breathing is more ragged, erratic, and labored.

6. *Notice how loud your breath is.* Efficient, diaphragmatic breathing is not loud. The deeper and more relaxed your breathing, the quieter it becomes. The breath quiets as it becomes increasingly effortless. *Effortlessness in breathing* is the clearest indication that you are breathing well.

FIVE PRINCIPLES FOR DEVELOPING DIAPHRAGMATIC BREATHING

Now that you have an initial sense of your breathing patterns, you can begin to improve them to reduce your pain. Keep in mind that diaphragmatic breathing is *easy* breathing. Learning diaphragmatic breathing is not about using specific breathing techniques, following specific rules, or having a breathing agenda. It is about learning *deeper bodily relaxation.*

If there is one thing you cannot force, it is relaxation. If you are a chest breather, you cannot *make* yourself breathe diaphragmatically and gain any benefit. If your breathing is short or ragged, or if it stops and starts, you cannot *force* yourself to breathe properly. Forcing brings tension into your body, and while you may feel you are breathing better if you force your breathing patterns to change, such changes will come only at the cost of tension.

To learn how to breathe diaphragmatically is to learn how to relax more deeply. After all, it is stress and tension that create pain, and it is by learning to release stress and tension that you reduce pain. Since you cannot simply decide to relax and breathe easily, you have to follow an indirect route: you have to coax the body into changing its habits, rather than forcing it to change. There are several principles that will help this process along. These principles are essential to all aspects of physical healing. While they are incorporated into the descriptions of the exercises below, being aware of them will help you work with those exercises more effectively. Absorb these principles now and refer to them frequently, and you will make swift progress.

1. *Observe and accept.* The best way to promote bodily relaxation is to observe and accept whatever your body is doing, rather than trying to change it. In the meditative breathing exercise that follows, you start by simply observing your breathing without judgment. You avoid trying to change it. In fact, you don't try to do anything. You don't try to follow the rules and be a good girl or good boy. You don't try to do things correctly. Instead, you allow yourself to experience what is actually happening in your body and, in particular, in your breathing. If you do this, your breathing will change on its own.

Nonjudgmental acceptance, rather than control, is the key to improvement and constructive change. Nonjudgmental acceptance promotes relaxation, which is why the breath deepens on its own if you observe it without interference. Your breathing gradually and steadily improves, becoming increasingly deep, open, and easy, simply by your noticing how it feels with an *interested, detached curiosity.*

2. *Focus on feeling your body rather than on doing something to it.* While nonjudgmental observation and acceptance are key to relaxation, this very process invites you to *feel* your breath and to *feel* your body. Feeling is synonymous with relaxation, and the more you feel your body with acceptance, the more its functioning automatically improves. Recall the story of Clara in chapter 1. Her numbness and pain dissipated as she worked at observing and accepting her body's sensations, learning how to feel without trying to control. This allowed her muscles to relax, her blood to flow, and her nerves to function more efficiently. Observation enhances feeling, and the ability to feel our bodies is a key element of any healing process. Our ability to feel corresponds to deeper relaxation.

Unfortunately, the chronic stress that plays a part in pain syndromes reduces our ability to feel because it brings tension into our bodies. The more tension we have, the less we can feel. On the other hand, the more we practice feeling, the less tension we will have.

Persons in chronic pain may think they are feeling too much rather than not enough. After all, they feel pain! Yet the pain they feel is frequently the result of being under too much tension for too long. The system finally breaks down because it has been unable to self-regulate by using feedback from its own sensations. Odd as it may seem, *pain is often the long-term result of a reduced ability to feel.* If you can decrease the tension in your body by feeling your body without reacting to or trying to control the sensations, you will eventually decrease the pain as well.

3. Imagine softness. The more we relax into feeling our breathing and our bodily sensations, the softer and more pliable our tissues become as they release unnecessary tensions and adhesions. Tense muscles are brittle and hard; relaxed muscles are pliable and soft. Using the imagination to enhance feelings of softness deepens your ability to release chronic tensions, open up your breathing, and quicken the process of pain reduction. The meditative breathing exercise that follows, as well as the numerous exercises in subsequent chapters, evoke images of softness to deepen bodily relaxation and neuromuscular release.

4. Practice kindness toward your body. When we have pain, we can become angry, disappointed, or frustrated with our body. This increases physical tension and also expresses an attitude of hostility and distrust toward our own flesh and blood. No one responds positively to hostility from others, and your body will not respond well to you if you adopt this attitude toward it. You and your body need to cooperate with each other if you are to improve the situation. Your body is part of you. Think of it as a sensitive child who needs love and attention. It needs to be listened to. Alternatively, think of your body as your partner in collaboration. To reach your goal, you must join together rather than stand in hostile camps.

Make a contract with your body to see it as your partner in healing.

Too many of us think of our bodies with displeasure, fear, or anxiety. We look at them critically. We tell ourselves we're too fat or too thin, too tall or too small, or too old. We don't like our neck or our shoulders or our digestion. We talk about our bodies as if they were betraying us. The problem is, we *are* our bodies. To heal, we have to recognize that we and our body are one—as science has indeed proven to be the case—and seek to work together, respecting the body's wisdom. The body is extremely sophisticated. It has far more to teach us than we imagine. Therefore, as you observe and work with your body, feel kindly and compassionately toward it. Assume an attitude of curiosity, attention, interest, and respect. It will reward you with improvements and an enhanced knowledge of yourself.

5. *Work with your breathing daily.* Because you are working to change habits of a lifetime that have resulted in chronic pain, you need patience and persistence. Habits change only through regular practice. The suggestions below are meant to be used on a daily basis until they become part of the way you automatically breathe. If you apply these suggestions regularly, then week by week, you will notice further incremental reductions in your level of pain. You will also develop insight about how to improve the quality of your life, a process that will further reduce pain.

Apply these five principles to working daily with the exercises below, and observe the beneficial results.

How to Develop Diaphragmatic Breathing

1. Practice Meditative Breathing

The meditative breathing exercise provides the foundation of all subsequent work, in this and subsequent chapters. This exercise teaches you how to relax deeply into the breath in a quiet, protective environment, free of distractions. It gives you the opportunity to focus your attention 100 percent on becoming aware of and gently transforming long-standing habits of breathing. Throughout the exercise, the combination of simple breath awareness and suggestive images opens and deepens the breath, in the process releasing unconscious muscle tensions that cause pain. It also reduces mental and emotional stress.

By practicing meditative breath awareness, most people become aware of a depth of relaxation, ease, focus, and self-awareness they have not experienced in years, if ever. Each time you work with it, the meditative exercise reduces tension, which has a ripple effect that carries through your day.

You should practice meditative breathing in a supportive, hassle-free environment in order to begin to heighten your body awareness, train your powers of self-observation, and change habitual breathing patterns. Use the meditative breathing exercise on a daily basis until you can breathe diaphragmatically: deeply, slowly, and easily. Achieving this goal may take anywhere from a few weeks to a few months. Give yourself the time to develop this invaluable skill!

To assist you in your practice, record the exercise described below on a tape, in a slow, gentle voice. Alternatively, you can order a cassette and/or CD I have created of this exercise, which includes musical accompaniment, through my Internet address, www.ingridbacci.com, or by sending your order through the mail, following the instructions on the order form on page 239.

Remember that meditative breathing is the foundation to your work with self-healing. Practice it every day, if possible.

Meditative Breath Exercise

1. *Find a quiet place.* Find a quiet place where you can lie down without interruptions for at least five and up to fifteen or twenty minutes. Make sure the phone is off and that your family knows this is your quiet time. Spend a few moments focused on your intention: to support yourself in finding greater tranquility.

2. *Scan your body.* With your eyes closed, gently scan your body with your attention. Start with your feet. Notice the way your toes, your heels, and the balls of your feet feel. Appreciate the sensations. There is no right or wrong here, just feeling. Take in the feeling of your ankles, calves, and thighs. Don't try to change anything. Be interested in the sensations, staying with them long enough to register them fully.

Continue like this up into your pelvis, abdomen, rib cage, shoulders, and neck. Take all the time you need to become fully present to the sensations of the different parts of your body.

Continue by scanning down your upper arms to your elbows, your lower arms, and then to your hands. Spend some time enjoying the feeling of the palms of your hands. They are full of nerve endings, and you may feel a tingling or warmth.

Now come to your face, and let yourself appreciate the softness of your lips. Once you have done this, move on to the area under your eyes, then to your cheeks, and then to your whole face. If you like, imagine that your face is like the face of a baby who is fast asleep: softer than the softest.

Once you have finished scanning the sensations of your limbs, torso, and head, let your awareness spread to include the feeling of your entire body.

Notice how the feeling of your body has changed. Do you feel it more clearly than when you started? Do you feel tingling or warmth? Do you feel heavy? Or light, as if you are floating? Do you feel bigger? These are typical relaxation responses.

3. *Feel your breath.* Now let your attention shift to the sensation of your breath as it moves in and out of your body. Put your hands over the area of your body where you feel your breath most clearly. It might be your chest, your diaphragm, or your belly. Let your attention rest on the feeling of your hands rising and falling as you breathe. As you focus on this sensation, you will notice thoughts going through your mind. Do not struggle with them or try to eliminate them. Let them be there, but come back to the feeling of your hands rising and falling with the breath, as if you are anchoring your attention in that sensation. Continue for a few minutes to focus on feeling your hands rising and falling with the breath.

4. *Feel the wave of the breath.* You will gradually become aware that the breath behaves in many ways like waves in the ocean. It simply flows in and out of you. Let yourself become absorbed in the feeling of the wave of the breath. If you were to get absorbed in watching waves hitting an ocean beach, you would become aware that each

wave is unique. One wave is powerful and strong, comes crashing down on the beach, and pulls out rapidly. The next wave is gentle and soft and lingers before withdrawing from the sand. Sitting there on the beach, you could drop into a fascinated trance absorbing how unique each wave is. Watch the breath in the same way. Appreciate how unique each breath is. Don't try to change it.

When you find yourself distracted by thoughts or feelings, gently bring your attention back to the feeling of the breath. You will gradually feel your entire body and mind becoming quieter and your breath becoming softer, slower, and deeper. Without effort, you are slipping into diaphragmatic breathing.

5. *Imagine that the breath is a caress.* Now imagine that the wave of the breath is like a caress coming into your body. Each wave reaches into you and caresses you on the inside. Because it is very soft, it invites you to open up and soften inside, to feel yourself more deeply. Feel how the caress of the breath touches you on the inside, inviting you to let down into feeling yourself. Feel that caress all the way into the area under your hands.

6. *Imagine the breath caressing you more deeply.* Once you have absorbed the sensation of the wave of the breath caressing the area under your hands, move your hands lower on your torso. If your hands were on your chest, they will now move toward your belly. If they were on your belly, they will move toward your pelvis. Again, *imagine* that the caress of the breath is now moving deeper into your body, into the area underneath your hands. Do not try to make your breath deeper. This will involve you in effort and control, which is counterproductive. Allow the imagination to do the work for you.

7. *Feel the breath filling your torso.* Continue the process of moving your hands down your body until you feel the breath easily and quietly filling your entire torso. Enjoy absorbing the feeling of open, deep breathing for as long as you like. Feel the internal pleasure this gives you.

Notice the changes in your body and mind. Is your breathing deeper? More relaxed? How does your body feel? Is your mind calmer? Did your mind jump around a lot at first, and is it quieter now? How do you feel emotionally? These changes are all part of learning deeper, easier, more meditative breathing.

8. *Open your eyes.* When you are ready to come to the close of your meditative breathing, open your eyes. See if you can maintain some awareness of the breath as you look around the room. When you get up, notice how present you can be to your breathing. Can you maintain some of the softness and depth of the breath that you have acquired? You are learning how to breathe diaphragmatically and reducing the physiological stress that contributes to pain.

9. *Repeat this exercise daily.* For the next month or more, repeat this meditative breathing exercise daily. You are retraining your breathing and learning how to relax deeply moment by moment. Once you know how to do this, you will no longer have to do the meditation each day. Instead, you will be incorporating its principles into your daily life.

2. Observe When You Hold Your Breath

The meditative breathing exercise asks you to set aside fifteen to twenty minutes each day to deepen your ability consciously to relax into breathing easily and diaphragmatically. This eliminates physiological stress and reduces chronic pain. Once you have practiced meditative breathing in your private space for a while, you will have learned enough breath awareness to take the next, very important step: to try to breathe more meditatively, or more diaphragmatically, *throughout* the day. We breathe all day, every day. It is *how* we breathe all day, every day, that creates stress and pain or freedom from stress and pain. As you work with yourself, it will be your breathing *throughout* the day that you gradually seek to influence through the breath awareness exercises provided in this chapter. Eventually, meditative or diaphragmatic breathing becomes not just a daily exercise of fifteen to twenty minutes duration but rather the way you breathe all the time.

I have developed a three-stage process to assist you in integrating breath awareness and meditative breathing into your daily life. While doing the meditative breath exercise requires a commitment of time on your part, none of the additional suggestions requires you to take time out of your day. After all, who has much time? More exercises can mean more stress, which is something you want to avoid. The following three suggestions simply ask you to observe how you are breathing at specific times and in specific activities and then to practice breathing more regularly, easily, and deeply at those times. Then observe the results.

The first of these additional suggestions is simply to *notice throughout the day when you hold your breath or breathe more shallowly than usual.* Many of us unconsciously bring tension into even the simple activities of daily living, such as washing dishes, talking, cooking, taking a walk, or driving a car. Once you start observing yourself, you may be surprised to discover that you hold your breath frequently, even every time you start moving!

One of my clients developed a clever way of reminding himself to notice his breathing patterns. For several months, he set the alarm on his digital watch to beep every forty-five minutes. He was frequently surprised, when the alarm beeped, to realize that he was breathing shallowly or holding his breath. Using the beeper alarm helped him become more aware, and as he became more aware, he changed his patterns, becoming more stress-free and relaxed.

To explore your breathing patterns, spend *one week* making a mental note of the situations in which you hold your breath. Notice your breathing when you change position; for example, when you get out of a chair, start walking, or bend over to pick something up. Also notice how you breathe when someone else is talking to you. Or when you are upset or angry. Or when you are under pressure. If you are like most people, you will notice that these situations often trigger an unconscious restriction in the body, a restriction that affects your breathing. You are in a subtle startle reflex that contributes to your pain.

When you find yourself breathing shallowly or holding your breath, avoid criticizing yourself for it. Self-criticism only brings further stress into your life, and that causes pain. Instead, congratulate yourself! You are making a leap in self-awareness that will help you reduce your pain.

When you notice yourself holding your breath or breathing shallowly, see if you can gently shift out of the habit. Can you breathe in a way similar to what you discovered in the meditative breathing exercise: softly, deeply, and quietly? Since you have been training yourself to open up your breathing, you will find that this is not too difficult. Notice how shifting your breathing affects you. Does it make it easier for you to do what you are doing? Does it reduce your tension or pain? Does it help you feel calmer or more focused? Keep track of how moving from holding your breath or breathing shallowly to breathing more deeply affects you throughout the day: physically, emotionally, and mentally.

You will know you are making real progress in following this suggestion when (a) you are far more conscious of the many times during the day that you may hold your breath; (b) you begin to reverse this habit and to breathe more regularly and deeply. Your goal is to move toward eliminating the tendency to restrict your breathing during the day. You are learning how to recognize and stop the pattern of restrictive breathing whenever it kicks in. The more you practice reversing the habit, the more you will be teaching your body to let go of physiological tension.

3. Breathe Consciously During a Simple Activity
One of the most efficient ways to make progress in changing breathing habits is to choose *one simple activity* and to make it your primary goal each day to (a) spend five to ten minutes being aware of how you breathe during this activity and (b) work gently on breathing more easily and deeply during this activity. The activity you choose should not require a lot of attention. It should be of low stress and of limited duration. Examples are: taking a shower, making your bed, watching the news on television, chopping vegetables for dinner, sitting at a table for a few minutes before eating, driving down the road, or taking a walk.

Why focus on breath awareness for a limited period of time while engaged in a simple, nonstressful activity? You may discover, by doing the meditative breathing exercise (exercise 1 above) and by observing when you hold your breath (exercise 2 above), that you can improve how you feel by deepening your breathing. Nonetheless, you will find it difficult to keep your breathing patterns in your awareness all day. After all, you have been breathing all your life without being mindful of how you breathe. Other things have been taking up your attention. Sometimes, how you are breathing is the furthest thing from your mind. Yet your breath is very important.

How, then, can you learn to be present to your breathing all the time? The best way to do this is to start small, by practicing breath awareness in limited time segments. Make it easy to focus on your breathing by doing this during activities that don't require a lot of concentration or trigger undue stress. Challenging situations tend to put us under greater stress, making it harder to learn the new skill of body release that is part of conscious breathing. The goal of breath training is to reduce stress, but the process of reaching that goal should start with mastering your breathing in less stressful rather than in more stressful situations.

In a five-to-ten-minute segment of each day, focus on breathing diaphragmatically during a nonstressful activity such as folding laundry, washing dishes, taking a walk, drinking your morning coffee or tea, making the bed, or clearing off your desk. To help you remember to do this, use the same activity each day. Let your attention focus on relaxing into your breathing. *Make breathing evenly and deeply more important than accomplishing your chosen activity.* This will teach you how to approach tasks from a foundation of physical and mental relaxation, rather than tension or anxiety.

At first, it may be a little difficult to stay with deep breathing. You may find that your breathing is quite restricted even while you perform simple activities, because stress has become a habit. Alternatively, you may find your attention repeatedly wandering away from your breath. Stay with your chosen simple activity until you begin spontaneously to be aware of breathing tensions and are able to correct them, and until you can stay consciously with your breath rather than letting your mind wander. As you breathe through your chosen activity, your stress will reduce; you will find the activity more pleasurable and your focus better. You will accomplish more, more easily.

Gradually, you will also find that you are spontaneously more aware of how you are breathing throughout the day and more able to shift into deeper, more relaxed breathing at will. You are making physiological relaxation rather than tension the basis of the way you approach your life. In the process, you are also discovering that relaxation is more efficient than tension.

4. Observe Your Breathing in More Challenging Situations

Once you can follow your breathing in simple daily activities, you will be able to follow your breathing and try to relax into diaphragmatic breathing in more challenging situations: a difficult conversation with a family member or friend, working at the computer, any stress-provoking situation. Give yourself time to develop this skill. You are trying to make easy breathing your *first* priority, so that you reduce the habitual tendency to react with stress to challenging situations. This reaction never helps you and only causes pain. The less you react to stress triggers, the more effective you will be and the less pain you will have. This does not mean suppressing your reactions to situations. It means learning how to calm yourself at deeper levels in the face of external stresses, so that those negative reactions do not even occur.

Notice how committing yourself to being more balanced in your breathing affects the situations in which you find yourself. How does breath awareness affect your interactions with people? Are you less reactive? How do others respond to you? Do they seem to feel more comfortable with you or to perceive you in a different way? In general, people find that the more they focus on breathing to induce physiological relaxation, even in the midst of stressful encounters, the less pain they feel, the more effective they are, the more others listen, and the less they react to tense situations.

RECOMMENDATIONS

As you practice these exercises, remember to use the five principles for deepening the breath and encouraging physiological relaxation. These are: (1) Observe and accept your breathing, no matter how it feels. Do not try to change it. It will change for the better on its own when you accept it. (2) Focus on *feeling* your body, rather than on *doing something* to it. (3) Imagine your body and breath as soft. This encourages deeper relaxation. (4) Adopt a kind, accepting, and friendly rather than critical attitude toward your body. (5) Practice breath awareness daily.

Because breath awareness work is such a vital foundation for pain reduction, you might consider joining a meditation group that works with it. Vipassana meditation is most likely to be of use to you in developing a calmer, deeper breath. You may also wish to read other books on breathing. Recommendations for further reading are included at the end of the chapter.

You will find it useful to keep a daily log of your progress in breath awareness until you have experienced so many of the benefits of breath awareness that you no longer need reminders to stay with your practice and it has become second nature. At the end of this chapter, you will find a daily log for your breathing exercises. Photocopy it and put it in a conspicuous place—on your fridge or bathroom mirror for instance—to help you stick with and observe your progress in breath awareness.

When you work with your breathing to heal from physical pain, you begin a process that has profound consequences: the process of listening to and collaborating with your body's feedback. You notice what makes your body feel calmer, more relaxed, and less effortful. You use this knowledge as a guide to help you feel better. This process of using bodily feedback has many levels, of which breath awareness is simply the first. You become aware of what your breathing feels like normally; then you explore how, by responding to your breathing in certain ways, your body relaxes more deeply, your muscle tension dissipates, and your pain recedes. By learning how to use your body's moment-by-moment feedback to guide it toward feeling better, you develop an important skill that most of us seriously underutilize.

By paying attention to your body's feedback, you begin to make your body's ease a *primary* focus of your attention rather than leaving it in the background. You make your body's relaxation and ease a priority under conditions where previously you tended to ignore it. You focus on breathing deeply even in situations that usually cause you to tighten up, and as a way to *reverse* those tension responses. You train yourself to feel less stress and pain by regularly focusing on self-calming. You become more efficient and feel more at ease.

By maximizing your own resources, your own ability to tune in to what feels better and worse for your body, and your ability to shift how you feel by getting in touch with breathing and with other techniques described in this book, you enhance your control over your body's health. You become your own researcher and, as far as possible, your own pain doctor. The key lies in listening to your body's wisdom and following its guidance to reduce tension throughout your body's tissues. Chapters 6 and 7 invite you to continue this process of listening to your body in order to reduce or eliminate chronic pain. In these chapters, you look at your alignment, at how misalignment fosters chronic pain, at the difference between what alignment and misalignment *feel* like, and at how to use this difference in feeling so as to reduce tension and pain. As in the chapters on breath awareness, improving alignment is not about following rules. It is about noticing how you can be more rather than less comfortable in your body. Improving your alignment is about doing things more easily.

Let's look next at what alignment is, what it isn't, and how it affects how we feel.

FURTHER READING

Joan Borysenko, *Minding the Body, Mending the Mind* (Reading, Mass.: Addison-Wesley, 1987). An early exploration of mind-body healing, including the use of meditation, by the former director of Harvard Medical School's Mind/Body Medical Institute.

Jon Kabat-Zinn, *Wherever You Go, There You Are* (New York: Hyperion, 1994). Useful and inspiring daily meditations by the founder and former director of the Stress Reduction Clinic at the University of Massachusetts Medical Center.

Daily Breath Awareness Log

1. Practice meditative breathing:
Today, _____ I did/_____ did not meditate for _____ minutes.

During and/or after meditation, I noticed that:
I was ___ more relaxed; ___ less relaxed.

My breathing ___ became deeper; _____ became slower;
___ didn't change.

I felt _____ emotionally or mentally calmer;
_____ didn't notice any change.

I noticed myself becoming more aware of some of my feelings
(please describe): _____

_____

_____.

I noticed that the meditation:
(a) __ helped me relax more during the day
(b) __ didn't affect the rest of my day.

2. Observe when you hold your breath:
Today, I noticed that I was holding my breath when

_____

_____

_____.

(Examples: getting up from a chair, standing, walking, washing
dishes, driving, talking to someone, etc.)

3. Breathe consciously during a simple activity:

Today, I practiced breathing consciously, regularly, and deeply in the following activity:

_____

_____.

(Examples: taking shower, reading, driving.)

I noticed that when I breathed consciously and deeply while doing this activity:

(a) __ I became more relaxed

(b) __ my pain bothered me less, or I felt less pain

(c) __ I tired less easily

(d) __ my concentration improved

(e) __ none of the above.

4. Observe your breathing in more challenging situations:

Today, I practiced staying with my breathing in the following challenging situation:_____

_____

_____.

I noticed that when I consciously relaxed into my breathing in this situation:

(a) __ my pain decreased

(b) __ I was less emotional

(c) __ I was more focused

(d) __ I could communicate better

(e) __ I could handle the situation better

(f) __ none of the above.

6

ALIGNMENT: A KEY TO FREEDOM OF MOVEMENT

Our bodies are remarkably complex machines, developed through thousands of years of evolution that fine-tuned our ability to move with speed, grace, and endurance. The ability to move easily and without pain, and to resist the strains of life effectively, is dependent on a subtle interaction of bones, joints, and muscles in which each partner performs a specific function. When the partners perform their proper functions, then muscles, bones, and joints tend to remain healthy. When one or more partners fail to perform their designated role, however, or take on work intended for the other partners, the body begins to suffer. If this situation persists for a long time, chronic pain results.

Our *bones* bear the primary responsibility for carrying our weight. When we stand correctly—which is synonymous with feeling relaxed, flexible, and mobile—our bones provide structural support. This leaves the joints free of pressure and enables them to work as hinges. It also offers the muscles the opportunity to relax and lengthen so they further support freedom in the joints and guide us through movement. When our bones perform their proper function, our bodies are said to be in alignment. When we are aligned, we feel comfortable.

When we are aligned, our bones *stack up* one upon the other. For example, when we stand aligned, the head rests directly on top of the spine, rather than jutting forward. When the head sits directly over the neck and the neck sits directly on top of the rest of the spine, the bones of the spine support the head and the neck muscles can relax. Similarly, when we are aligned, our back is straight rather than hunched or swaybacked, our shoulders, hips, knees, and feet are all neatly stacked in a vertical line, and our weight is distributed evenly on both feet. Bone supports bone.

When we are not aligned—for example, when our head and neck jut forward and our neck and back muscles have to work to hold the head up, or when we lean forward or back, hunch or collapse, tilt to one side, and so on—this puts pressure on the joints, contributing to arthritis, disc degeneration, tearing of cartilage, and joint and membrane inflammation. In addition, *the muscles must now carry the weight of the body. They do this by bracing and contracting.* When muscles contract too often for too long, they become chronically tight and painful. They also put further pressure on bones and joints. This physiological stress initiates a cycle of chronic muscle pain, joint pain, inflammation, and arthritis. Muscles are meant for movement and to maintain space between the joints. They are not meant to carry our weight. This is why misalignment—the failure of the bones to carry the weight of the body—is a major source of chronic pain. *A characteristic of all forms of misalignment is excess muscle tension.* Where exactly the muscles carry excess tension depends on the type of misalignment.

What Causes Misalignment?

Accidents and genetic factors can contribute to misalignment, but *the single most important cause of misalignment is the way we use our bodies.* Think of how many hours you spend each day sitting in a chair. Perhaps you lean on one hip more than the other, hunch forward, or crane your head as you work at your desk and stare into the computer screen. Perhaps when you stand, you unwittingly lean forward or back or stand with your weight primarily on one leg. Perhaps when you work out at the gym, you lean a little bit to one side as you push through the resistance of the weights with which you are working. Such seemingly insignificant variations in stance take us out of alignment. They increase the effort expended by muscles and the pressure felt by joints. They cause physiological stress. Over time, these habits play a substantial role in the development of pain syndromes.

Improper habits of walking can also be a source of misalignment. The average person walks 8,000 steps a day, or approximately 75,000 miles, by the age of fifty. If we spend years walking out of alignment, the body inevitably cries out in pain.

For thousands of years, and until as recently as a hundred years ago, most people lived close to nature and developed proper alignment. Unfortunately, many factors in the environment today contribute to poor alignment: our sedentary lifestyle, the harsh impact on our bodies of cement walkways and soft sofas, crowded spaces, the constrained sitting postures imposed on us by long hours of sitting at the computer or at desk jobs, overuse of cars and underuse of our legs to get us around, an exercise technology that encourages people to use exercise machines on a one-size-fits-all model, and general lack of public knowledge of good principles of body use.

We live in a largely artificial world that imposes its own unforgiving rules on the body. We lack movement in our lives, and we lack the variety of physical tasks that fosters spontaneous and natural alignment. Each of us must therefore consciously learn the principles of alignment and movement that once came spontaneously. If you want to have healthy bones, joints, and muscles, you must learn how to use your body's feedback consciously to develop healthy alignment. The result will be both a reduction in pain and an increase in your feeling of ease, grace, and vitality.

While environmental factors contribute to poor body use and misalignment, emotional and mental stress also play a major role. We all instinctively recognize the postural stances of persons under stress. Often these stances become habitual. A man who deals with the tension of stress through aggression may have a jutting jaw, musclebound shoulders, and a stiff walk, while his fear-based colleague may have a collapsed abdomen, sunken shoulders, and forward-jutting head. Women can, of course, manifest the same patterns. They may also adopt more culturally sanctioned feminine ways of exhibiting postural stress in their bodies: a tense neck, jutting bust, and overly bright eyes; or a depressed, sunken, and burdened posture. As author Stanley Keleman points out in his book *Emotional Anatomy*, the various muscle-tensing expressions of the startle reflex all compromise our alignment. Learning to let go of those postural expressions of disempowerment reduces stress and pain while enhancing self-esteem.

How Can You Improve Your Alignment?

Most people are not aware of when their bodies are misaligned. The way they use their bodies is habitual, and habits are generally unconscious. We don't think about the way we stand, sit, and walk. We just do these things the way we have always done them. Too often, the way we have always done them is stressful to us. What's more, habits have a way of perpetuating themselves. They feel right simply because they are familiar. Unfortunately, what is familiar can all too often become the source of pain.

As you work with correcting your alignment, you will be moving from the familiar to the unfamiliar. At first, the unfamiliar will feel a little weird and strange. But you will soon find that it also feels better. *All improvements in alignment reduce the level of effort in the body.* Your guide to improving alignment will therefore involve noticing areas of effort and tension in your body and using techniques to reduce that tension and effort. You will be letting go of long-standing habits of physical stress.

When you have chronic pain, you tend to use more effort in everyday activities than persons who are free of pain. Yet you are not generally aware of this. If you knew you could do things with less effort, clearly you would! Consequently, as you go through the principles described in this chapter, and the tools for improving alignment described in chapter 7, you will be discovering where you use more effort than necessary. Simultaneously, you will be learning to let go of that effort.

Learning alignment is an art in many disciplines. Within the field of chronic pain reduction, the most famous is the Alexander Technique. Founded by Frederick Matthias Alexander in the mid–twentieth century, the Alexander Technique has become world-famous as a tool for reducing chronic pain and enhancing fluidity and grace. Today, the Alexander Technique is utilized both as an adjunct to physical therapy and traditional medical treatment, and in dance and musical performance schools and institutes throughout the world. Other highly effective movement approaches to learning better alignment include Aston Patterning and many of the martial arts.

Proper alignment can reduce chronic pain and enhance peak athletic performance. This book cannot give you a full training in alignment, but the principles and exercises offered here will provide you with some highly useful, specific tools for reducing pain in daily activities. They will also give you essential awareness techniques that you can apply to numerous situations to continue to improve your alignment. Keep these principles in mind, make them second nature, and you will move more easily.

Chapter 7 demonstrates how to use a series of simple awareness exercises to improve your alignment while standing, sitting, and walking. You will gain the greatest benefit from these exercises if you pay attention to the four principles below.

FOUR PRINCIPLES FOR IMPROVING ALIGNMENT

1. Notice your habits. As you go through the self-awareness exercises in chapter 7, begin by paying attention to how you ordinarily do things: for example, where you carry your weight on your feet, how you sit in a chair, what muscles you use to move from sitting to standing. You will bring unconscious tension habits to light. The more aware you are of what your body is doing and how it differs from what it does when it is better aligned, the more quickly you will be able to replace habits that cause pain with habits that reduce pain.

2. Focus your interest on how, not on what. When you want to cross the room, sit down, or pick up a book, you don't generally pay attention to how you are doing these movements. You just focus on the end result, on what you want to accomplish. This is a major reason pain becomes a problem: you are not paying attention to what your body is telling you about levels of tension you are carrying; you are not giving this information priority; and you are not using your sensori-motor feedback. A good driver uses his or her car's responses to gauge when to shift gears, and how quickly to brake. We drive our own cars—our bodies—without adequate attention to their responses. To develop good alignment, you have to pay as much attention to how you are moving as to what you are trying to accomplish by moving.

An infant learns to crawl, sit, stand, and walk by listening to his own bodily feedback and continually finding the easiest, least effortful way to move. Evolution has created us so that when we pay attention to our body, the easiest movement is the right movement. A baby innately understands this. A good athlete learns how to hit a tennis serve better, or drive a golf ball off the tee better, by paying attention to the feeling of his body and learning how to work with more precision, greater ease, and less effort. Most of us fail to do that, even though we may watch someone participating in a sport, playing a musical instrument, or running down the street, and realize that she would perform much better if she dropped her shoulders or relaxed her arms.

We are often so focused on where we want to walk that we fail to notice that we are leaning forward or holding our arms rigidly as we walk. Or we are focused so intently on getting information we need off the Internet that we fail to notice that our body is collapsed into the chair and our head is leaning way forward. Because we are concentrating on *what* and ignoring *how*, our bodies suffer. To learn to change inefficient habits of alignment, you have to stop focusing on what you want to get done and start focusing on how you are using your body and on whether you could change how you are using your body so as to reduce the effort you expend.

Focusing on how you do things requires slowing down, being patient, and letting go of your focus on the goal. Let yourself truly explore subtle shifts in movement in the exercises that follow. Pay attention above all to how you feel as you do the exercises. A feeling of relative effort corresponds to tension. A feeling of relative ease corresponds to muscular release. Give your body plenty of time to experience the new movement patterns.

3. *Follow the principle of ease.* There is only one reason to improve your alignment: *it feels better!* Often, we approach exercises with a sense of duty and work, but the alignment exercises you will explore are not about work. They are about decreasing the work you are already doing by helping your body to move more efficiently. The exercises are also not about doing things the "right" way. They are about doing things in a way that feels easier and better. The subjective sensations that accompany a decrease in workload are pleasure, relaxation, and ease. These are your body's feedback indicating that you are improving the way you are living in your body. Listen to your feedback, and ignore notions you may have about the correct way to do things. Let your body be king, and, as you do this, let yourself follow the principle of ease. When your movement feels more relaxed and limber, you will know you are on the right path.

4. *Breathe throughout.* Remember that diaphragmatic breathing is integral to proper alignment. When your breathing is shallow, you tend to use your muscles rather than your bones to support your weight, and this causes misalignment. When you breathe fully, you automatically improve your alignment. Pay attention to your breathing as you do the exercises, and try to keep it deep, easy, and relaxed. Breathing and alignment enhance each other: the better you breathe, the more aligned you are, and the better your alignment, the more easily you breathe.

In chapter 7, you will learn how to apply these four principles to three activities we perform every day: standing, sitting, and walking.

FURTHER READING

Frederick Matthias Alexander, *The Use of the Self* (New York: E. P. Dutton, 1932). The philosophy behind the Alexander Technique, written by its founder and with an introduction by the American philosopher John Dewey.

Michael Gelb, *Body Learning* (New York: Henry Holt, 1981). An excellent, very readable introduction to the concepts of the Alexander Technique.

7

FINDING YOUR WAY TO
EFFORTLESS ALIGNMENT

We stand, sit, and walk every day. If you can improve your alignment and efficiency in these activities, you will go a long way toward reducing your pain. Following the recommendations below, remember to use the four principles described in chapter 6. Please use the log at the end of this chapter to keep a record of your progress in improving the way you stand, sit, and walk. Make a copy of the log and put it in a conspicuous place to remind yourself about alignment awareness, until your awareness has become second nature. Remember that regular practice of the principles of healthy alignment alters stressful physical habits of a lifetime and provides substantial rewards.

IMPROVE YOUR ALIGNMENT WHEN STANDING

I discovered how important the way we stand is for how we feel through my own personal experience. For about fifteen years, starting at the age of thirty-three, I suffered from chronic pain.

Because I was unable to find medical help that alleviated my condition, I spent a great deal of time exploring my body. This gave me a deep personal understanding of how the body works and eventually led to a healing that was so complete that, twenty-five years later, I remain in peak physical condition, enjoy great vitality, and am blessed to be able to participate freely and with joy in numerous athletic activities. My present good health is a direct result of numerous small realizations that changed the way I viewed and lived in my body. One of these many realizations had to do with the way I stood.

On one of those typical days when my back gnawed with discomfort, I had a minor epiphany. I was standing in a crowded New York City subway car, on my way to work. My low back was killing me! I shifted around a bit, and some instinct told me to unlock my knees and bend them. I noticed that bending my legs just a little bit seemed to ease the stress on my back. And so whenever I had to stand for long periods of time—on the subway, in a grocery store, at a reception—I would notice whether my knees were locked, something that I had never been conscious of before. Then I would bend my legs just enough to soften at the knees. Invariably, I felt better. I also realized I could focus more effectively on whatever task I was engaged in, since the pain no longer absorbed my attention.

This experience encouraged me to look more closely at what I was doing with my legs that might be contributing to my chronic pain. The self-observation yielded all sorts of information about habits I had of which, like most people, I was completely unaware. For example, I realized that I tended to stand on my left leg and to put my right leg out to the side. I had probably developed this habit because one leg is slightly longer than the other. Like any habit, it felt familiar and therefore right. But when I looked at myself in the mirror, I saw that carrying most of my weight on my left leg resulted in my pelvis having a marked tilt. That tilt could be contributing to my pain, and I started trying to change my pattern and put my weight equally into both legs. After having spent thirty years standing more on one leg than on the other, that was difficult, but I noticed that if I did so consistently, my back felt better and seemed to go into spasm less frequently. I also noticed that I felt more personally secure and focused. Subtle emotional and mental changes accompanied slight shifts in body posture.

What we do with our legs plays a critical role in how the rest of us feels. Our legs are our foundation. They are meant to offer a solid support to the rest of our bodies and to our minds. When we let our legs do the job of carrying our weight, our torso feels more relaxed, and we feel tired less easily. Find this out for yourself by exploring the following suggestions. Notice how they help reduce fatigue and pain when you stand.

1. *Notice how you stand.* Stand the way you normally do and observe yourself. Pay careful attention, and be sure to answer all the following questions to your own satisfaction.

a. Are your knees locked, or are they slightly bent?
b. Is your weight evenly distributed over both legs, or are you standing more on one leg than the other?
c. How far apart are your feet?
d. Is the distance between your feet greater than, less than, or the same as the distance between your hips?
e. Are your feet turned out, turned in, or facing straight forward?
f. Is your weight more on the balls of your feet, more on the heels, or evenly distributed between front and back?
g. Is your weight more on the inside of your feet, more on the outside of your feet, or balanced between the inside and the outside?

Make a note of everything you have observed before going on to the next steps.

Many people stand with their knees pulled back or locked, which creates problems. It gives a false sense of stability, because the legs become rigid, and it stresses the knee joints. Locked knees also cause the pelvis to tilt forward, putting pressure on the hips, which can cause hip pain. The forward tilt of the pelvis also creates a swayback. You can easily observe this swayback if you stand sideways in front of a mirror and alternate between locking and unlocking your knees. A swayback puts the entire spine out of alignment and causes muscles in the low back, neck, and shoulders to overwork in order to support the spine, leading to pain in those areas and eventually even to spinal degeneration.

Once you have observed your own pattern of standing, follow the recommendations below to improve your alignment and your sense of ease.

2. *Unlock your knees.* By unlocking your knees, you automatically move your pelvis and hips into better alignment and reduce unnecessary pressure on the muscles. To unlock your knees, simply bend them very slightly and gently. If you initially feel less stable in doing this, be aware that this is because you are used to associating stability with rigidity. The feeling of instability will soon pass, to be replaced by a sense of greater balance.

Make a point of noticing, when you are standing talking to a friend or waiting in line at the grocery store, whether your knees are locked or free. When you notice that your knees are locked, simply unlock them. You will begin to find standing less tiring.

3. *Align your feet.* Are your feet turned out when you stand? Many people stand with their feet turned out too far. Unfortunately, this contributes to a swayback, stressing your back, shoulders, and neck. Standing with your feet turned out also tends to round your shoulders and compress your chest. Rounded shoulders set the stage for rotator cuff and tennis elbow injuries, as well as a host of other arm, shoulder, and upper back problems. A compressed chest makes breathing difficult and compromises not only the lungs but also the heart and digestive functions. If you stand with your feet turned out, your ankles probably pronate as well, leaning inward and destroying the structural stability of your foundation joint. If your ankles aren't stable, everything above them suffers. Turned-out feet can create knee and hip pain, neck problems, and headaches.

How does the distance between your feet affect you? If your natural foot stance is wider or narrower than the width of your hips, your legs will not be directly underneath you and therefore will not give you adequate support. See what it feels like to stand with your feet four to eight inches apart, with the toes just slightly turned out and the heels only marginally closer to each other than the toes, so that they line up with the middle of the hip joint. When your heels are directly under the middle of your hip joint, you have maximum support, your ankles are stable, and your back is better aligned. If you are not used to this stance, give yourself time to adjust. Make smaller adjustments initially, and then build over time. This will give unused muscles time to adapt to the new load-bearing requirements.

4. *Redistribute the weight over your feet.* What did you notice about where you carry your weight on your feet? Are you more on the balls or the heels, or neither? Do you stand more on the inside or the outside of your feet, or neither? When your weight is properly distributed over your feet, *it is evenly distributed both between the two feet and between the front and back of each foot.* The weight also falls more to the outside rather than the inside of the foot. Standing with the weight more on the balls of your feet contributes to locked knees, a swayback, and compressed joints. Standing with the weight more on the heels compresses the front of the body and reduces support. Carrying the weight on the inside of the foot instead of the outside makes the ankles pronate (collapse inward), putting pressure on the ankles and knees, a pressure that inevitably travels up through the entire spine and torso. Standing with your weight on the inside of your feet can create foot pain and lead to herniated cervical discs.

To explore what it feels like to balance your weight evenly between the front and back of your feet, rock gently forward and backward, bending at the ankle joints and keeping the rest of your body straight. Let your whole body hinge from the ankles, but do not lock your knees. As you rock forward and backward, gradually make this motion smaller and smaller, until you feel that you can identify the midpoint where your weight is evenly distributed between the front and back of your feet. This is the neutral point of alignment. Absorb how this feels, so that you can remember the feeling during the day and improve your standing pattern.

Now explore how to distribute your weight evenly between your feet. Rock sideways gently, once again initiating the movement at your ankles, so that your hips and torso do not get involved. Gradually make the movements smaller until you can feel the weight evenly between your two feet.

Once you have balanced the weight between your two feet and between the front and back of your feet, can you also rest your weight more on the outside than the inside of your feet? Your weight is now evenly distributed between your two legs and between the front and back of your feet. Absorb the sensation.

Notice throughout the day how well your weight is distributed over your feet, and gently correct any imbalance when you find it. Gradually, this self-correction will become automatic. Your new posture will contribute to your feeling more energetic and less easily fatigued when you stand. Learning to stand balanced over your feet can avert years of discomfort—an amazingly small action to reap such a large benefit!

5. *Feel the weight of your body in your legs by grounding.* When you allow the bones of your legs to carry the full weight of your body, your weight transfers through your legs and down into the earth. This is commonly called being "grounded." The more grounded we feel, the easier it is to stand. When we are not well grounded, we use muscular effort to hold ourselves up, rather than allowing the relationship between our bones and the earth to give us full support. When we hold ourselves up, we develop upper body tension, raised shoulders, neck and back pain, and even knee pain. *Lack of grounding is a very common cause of pain.*

To ground your weight through your legs, try the following exercise of your imagination: Stand fully relaxed, with your eyes closed to eliminate distractions. Imagine that your feet are growing roots into the ground. Let those roots grow very deep. Extend those roots as far below the ground as you are tall, whether that is five feet, six feet, or more. Feel the support those roots offer you. As you do this, you will automatically release tension from your torso and allow your bones to carry you more efficiently.

This reduction in tension may initially feel unfamiliar, even weird. Your torso may feel lighter and your legs heavier. Your body may feel like swaying, as a tree feels free to sway in the wind because it is well supported by its roots. Initially, this swaying sensation may feel un-nerving, but it also has a very positive effect: it activates your internal balancing mechanisms. When you can sway, rather than standing rigid, you are like the bamboo tree, whose flexibility has inspired Eastern philosophers and healers to use it as a symbol of strength. If you accustom yourself to the sensation of grounding, which makes you strong and supple without being rigid, you will find that your back, shoulders, and neck relax considerably and you will suffer less from fatigue. This is because your legs, rather than your torso, are doing the work of carrying your weight.

One of my clients was training for her black belt in karate. She fo-cused on grounding through her standing leg while kicking with her other leg. She found that this gave her much greater power and con-trol. Because she was firmly anchored through her standing leg, she could kick more powerfully with the other leg. Another client whose job required her to speak in front of large audiences used the ground-ing technique when lecturing. The grounding not only reduced her back pain in that high-stress job but also bred in her a sense of confi-dence and personal authority. On a physiological level, she was con-sciously reversing the startle reflex, which kicks in under situations of stress. The tightening involved in the startle reflex tends to pull us up out of our legs and into our neck and shoulders, creating a lot of ten-sion in the upper body. Because this client reversed her startle reflex by focusing attention down in her body, she was better able to *stand her ground*.

Like most of the breath awareness exercises, the tools just described for improving the ease of standing take no time out of your day. They simply ask you to give a bit more attention to how you are in your body as you stand in various activities.

IMPROVE YOUR ALIGNMENT WHEN SITTING

During the years when I suffered from chronic back pain, getting out of a chair was often a painful ordeal. When sitting down, I also frequently felt stiff and awkward. I never thought of this problem as something over which I could establish conscious control; instead I told myself that I had a bad back and there was nothing to be done about it. That changed when I took my first lesson in the Alexander Technique. The practitioner asked me to move from sitting to standing a few times. As she watched, I obeyed—with difficulty and pain. Then, using her hands and making verbal suggestions, she took me through some slight adjustments that initially seemed inconsequential. She helped me shift the position of my legs, back, and neck, had me bend from the hips rather than the waist, and—all of a sudden—I was out of the chair and free of pain! Then we reversed the movement, and she helped me get back into the chair, again using touch and verbal guidance. I felt more graceful and fluid than I had in years.

This experience was the beginning of my awareness that the way I moved from sitting to standing, and from standing to sitting, was playing a big part in creating the pain in my back, hips, knees, shoulders, and neck. It also taught me that *pain results from using too much effort*. The Alexander Technique lessons helped me notice unconscious muscular effort in the muscles of my torso. They also taught me how to inhibit that effort and tension and to move more freely.

Below you will find a simple set of procedures that you can follow to go from sitting to standing and back to sitting with less effort. This process will greatly reduce discomfort if you have pain in these movements as a result of excessive physiological stress. It will also contribute to better alignment and body mechanics. If you wish to use audiovisual supports to learn how to move more fluidly from standing to sitting and back to standing, the steps described below are in my video and DVD program, *Reduce Your Chronic Pain*, which you can order through my Web site, www.ingridbacci.com, or by following the ordering instructions at the end of this book.

To learn how to move more easily between sitting and standing, start with self-observation. Remember that you will be paying attention to how your body and in particular your *torso* feel as you experiment. You will be looking for a sense of reduced effort in the torso.

Proper sitting is not about following a set of rules; it is about finding out what feels easier and more efficient.

Let's start by looking at one of the key components in going from sitting to standing and back to sitting: bending.

1. *Observe how you bend.* Bend over from a standing position, as if you were about to sit down in a chair, but don't sit down fully. Notice how you make this bending motion. Take the time to repeat this motion as often as you need and to answer each of the following questions: Where do you feel the work in your body? Pay close attention. Do you feel any tension in your back, neck, or shoulders? Are your abdominal muscles working? Are you holding your breath? If you answer "Yes" to any of these questions, as 99 percent of people do, then you are overusing muscles in your torso. They are doing work they were not meant to do.

Now observe closely whether your torso is straight or curved as you bend over. You may want to position yourself sideways in front of a full-length mirror to obtain an accurate impression. If you bend from the hip joints, your torso is more likely to be straight. If you bend from the waist, or if you pull your head back while bending, your torso will be curved rather than straight. When it curves, whether in flexion or in extension, it goes out of alignment. Now observe how much your knees and hips bend. Make a note of everything you observe.

When we bend easily, as nature meant us to do, our entire torso stays uninvolved in the movement and feels totally relaxed. In addition, rather than curving, it forms a single straight line from the top of our head to our tailbone. When the torso does not participate in the bending motion—and this is the ideal—we feel *no tension* or muscular contraction in our abdomen, neck, shoulders, or back, and our breath is full and deep. To bend without stress, we need to *fold over at our joints* rather than use our torsos, and there should be maximum freedom and range of motion within the joints. To explore how to bend efficiently and effortlessly, follow the directions below.

2. *Bend from the hips.* Our hip joints are the most important joints in the body. We must use them properly if we are to move with-

out effort or stress. Yet most people use their hip joints far too little. You may not even know where your hip joints are. To find them, sit down with your buttocks close to the front of your chair and both feet flat on the floor. Put the fingertips of each hand in the crease between your thighs and your pelvis. You are contacting the front of your hip joints. Now rock gently forward and back over these joints, keeping your torso straight and allowing *all the movement* to originate at the hinge formed by the hip joints.

Again, it will help you to have a mirror to observe your movement. You will know you are moving correctly when your back feels relaxed and your body tilts forward and backward easily. As you pivot forward, your head will be looking straight down at the floor. As you come back up, your head will return to a position where you are looking forward. Notice that bending from the hip joints eliminates all effort from the muscles of your torso and helps keep the bones of your spine aligned.

3. *To bend from a standing position, use both the hip and knee joints.* When you bend to go from standing to sitting, you bend by adding another element. You bend at *both* the hip *and* the knee joints, while keeping your torso uninvolved. Many people bend either at the hips alone or at the knees alone. This creates stress for the back, which you can readily feel if you try bending from a standing position by folding over either only at the hip joints or only at the knees. Be sure, therefore, to bend as much as possible at *both* joints. Stand up and practice bending by folding simultaneously at both the knees and the hip joints. You are moving in the direction of a squat, with the addition that as you go into your squat, your torso approximates a position that is *horizontal*. You will look a little bit like a sprinter in the starting box, except that your head will be facing the floor and your eyes will be looking at the floor.

To come back to standing, straighten at the knees and hips. Do not forget to breathe throughout this movement, since the moment you stop breathing, you will be tightening muscles in your torso.

You will know you are doing this movement correctly, and experiencing greater ease in bending, when you feel no tension or effort in your torso—your neck, shoulders, back, or abdomen. Your legs will be doing the work, and your body will be pivoting over its hip and knee joints.

4. *Shift your weight back on your heels to bend and forward on the balls of your feet to stand.* Bending to sit becomes even easier when you initiate it by letting your weight shift back on your heels before you bend. Similarly, initiate returning to an upright position by shifting forward onto the balls of your feet before you straighten up. Practice rocking slightly back on the heels to bend and then rocking forward on the balls of your feet to go from bending to standing. Repeat this movement several times. See how easy it becomes!

You can now incorporate what you have learned about bending into getting effortlessly into and out of a chair.

5. *Bend fully to sit down.* To practice sitting down, place a chair directly behind you, so that you are almost touching it with the back of your legs. Now, without looking at the chair, initiate bending: rock back onto your heels, bending fully at both the hip joints and knees while breathing easily and letting your entire torso move as a single unit. As you bend forward, you are simulating a squat, with your torso almost horizontal with the floor and your head facing the ground, rather than looking out in front of you. Keep on bending at both the hips and the knees—like an accordion—until your bottom touches the chair. You don't have to look behind you to find the chair. Your buttocks will find it. You will be surprised to find that bending into a squat this way makes sitting easy. That's because you are bending the way nature meant you to, using your joints to fold your body over onto itself, and keeping your torso free of effort. If you are accustomed to using your arms for support when getting into a chair, you'll find you do not need to do this. Your arms can just hang by your sides.

Why does sitting become so easy when done this way? Because you are using your legs and joints to do the work, and your torso is staying relaxed. Since your torso was never meant to engage in the work of bending or sitting, you are no longer abusing it. Everything works better.

6. To go from sitting to standing, bend fully. To move effortlessly from sitting to standing, you must sit as far forward as possible in your chair and place your feet flat on the ground, as close to the chair as possible and as much underneath you as you can manage. By doing this, when you bend forward, *your weight will be directly over your feet.* Now, while continuing to sit, pivot all the way forward at the hip joints, breathing easily and keeping your back and neck in a single line. You will know you are doing this correctly if you feel *no* muscle tension in your neck, shoulders, back, or abdomen and your eyes end up looking at the floor. If you are far enough forward in the chair, and if your feet are as far underneath you as they can be, your weight will be directly over your feet, your torso will be almost horizontal, and you will have excellent leverage for using only your legs to get you out of the chair. To rise to standing, *inhale deeply,* and, while inhaling, push down through your feet into the floor and . . . you're up! If you have used only your feet and legs to push you from sitting to standing, your torso will feel totally relaxed and standing up will feel effortless, with the exception of the work done by your legs. As with sitting down, you will find that there is no need to use your arms when you let your legs and feet do the work.

Once again, the key to reducing muscle tension in your body is to *let your legs and feet do the work,* while engaging the joints of your hips and knees to bend. *Use your torso less. Use your legs and joints more.* Though you might think that using your joints more would increase your hip or knee pain, the opposite is the case. Hip and knee pain tend to be the result of long-term inefficient use of the muscles attached to these joints, rather than problems inherent in the joints themselves. Except in extreme cases of long-term degeneration of the joints, using your joints correctly will tend to correct muscle imbalances that contribute to joint dysfunction. This will reduce pain.

IMPROVE YOUR ALIGNMENT WHEN WALKING

When we see people walking down the road at a distance, we spontaneously and intuitively evaluate their relative age, even if we cannot see their face, from the way they walk. If they move slowly, with little spring to their feet and little swing in their bodies, we assume they are older. If they move fluidly, with a spring to their feet and their arms and torso swinging freely, we assume they are younger.

Our quality of movement corresponds to our biological age—to how well we have weathered time—while our chronological age often shows in our face.

So accustomed are we to evaluating someone's age by the quality of his or her movement that we tend to think that being older *means* having a stiffer, more rigid, and less bouncy walk and being younger *means* having more spring and flexibility in your walk. But this equation is far from accurate. It would be more accurate to turn it around and say that the less limber you are in your walk, the older, more infirm, and more pain-ridden you become in your body, whereas the more limber you are in your walk, the younger, livelier, and more healthy you become in your body. Putting it this way has two implications: first, that the quality of your gait is not something that inevitably deteriorates with age but is within your control; and second, that the quality of your gait has a lot to do with whether or not your body hurts. By working to change the quality of your gait, you can go a long way toward both decreasing your pain and increasing your freedom of movement.

When I was in my thirties, I walked with great difficulty and looked old. As I write this book, at least once a week someone tells me that I look fifteen years younger than my chronological age and that I walk with the spring of a young woman. My body got younger as I became older after I became aware of how I walked, realized that the way I was walking was making me older, stiffer, and more sore, and learned to use my body's feedback to walk more easily and effortlessly. The more I reduced the effort or muscular tension of walking, the better my body felt.

I recently witnessed a dramatic transformation in a woman who was attending one of the chronic pain management classes I teach for the HMO Oxford Health Plans. She came into this particular seminar late. At the break, she approached me and lamented bitterly that she had constant back pain. She had just come from yet another visit to the doctor, who had told her there was nothing more that he could do for her. I told her how sorry I was to hear this and expressed the hope that the day's class would help her.

The focus of the class was on learning how to walk with less effort and more ease. At the end of the day, this woman came up to me smiling broadly. Much of her pain had dissipated that day, simply by her learning how to change the way she walked—even though her doctor had told her that very day that her case was beyond repair! The next class, after she had practiced walking for a week, she returned to the seminar and told the entire class what a difference changing her manner of walking had made in her life.

A sleep-deprived mom who worked with me on walking more easily and gracefully relayed the effect that walking awareness had made in her life on a more personal level. Her infant son woke her frequently during the night, and her habit had been to tromp tiredly over to his crib to pick him up. After working with me, this mom began to notice how she walked during her midnight labors: with a heavy, stiff tread. She decided to walk more consciously and to follow the guidelines I had given her. She noticed that this affected her attitude toward her son: "When I practiced walking with more spring, I felt less exhausted, more alive, and more present to my son. Even though nighttime feedings can be difficult, I enjoyed them more."

Learning how to stand and sit more easily involves using your legs and feet more, while simultaneously reducing the work of the muscles of your torso: your neck, shoulders, back, and abdomen. In learning how to walk more effortlessly, you will continue this process. You will learn how to reduce the tension in your torso and to use your legs and feet more efficiently. Begin with some self-observation:

1. *Observe how you walk.* Take a short walk, and notice what this feels like.

   a. Does it feel effortful? Do you feel *any tension at all* in your neck, shoulders, back, abdomen, hips, or knees?

b. Are you breathing easily? Do you find yourself holding your breath, breathing shallowly, or breathing in a broken rhythm?

c. Observe your foot strike. Do your feet face straight forward when you walk, or do they turn out? Does one foot turn out more than the other?

d. As you shift weight from one leg to the other in walking, do you push off through the ball of your foot or more from the side of your foot or your big toe?

e. Do you have a clear heel/toe action, or do you land more on the whole of your foot?

f. Is there a bounce in your walk or not? Do you shuffle?

> *Fully observe all these aspects of your walking. Make a note of what you have discovered.*

Many people breathe shallowly when they walk. They also carry a fair amount of tension in their neck, shoulders, arms, back, or abdomen. These are all signs of excess muscular effort and holding, all of which can in turn create anything from headaches to shoulder or back pain to hip, knee, or foot problems. This excess tension reflects the fact that the torso is working too hard and that the legs and feet, which are meant to support the torso, are working too little and inefficiently. A major reason for this is that the flat, hard surfaces of our cement-covered world discourage us from using our legs and feet the way we should.

Imagine yourself back in nature. In this body-friendly environment, the uneven and softer quality of the ground would be compelling you continually to use the joints and muscles of your feet to find a good footing, and you would learn to rely on the flexibility and responsiveness of your legs and feet to move you through space. In the process, you would shift your weight actively from one leg to the other and use your feet agilely, perhaps a bit like your ancestors, the tree-dwelling primates. To use another analogy, your feet and ankles would act something like the shock absorbers of a car, cushioning your torso from their impact with the ground.

For your feet to operate as shock absorbers, they have to have spring and flexibility. As you walk or run through uneven territory, you also have to shift your weight easily and fully from one leg to the other to keep your balance. When the feet and legs act this way, the torso can swing freely above them, fully relaxed. But none of this happens in our urban environment. Unyielding sidewalks and floors, combined with stiff shoes that don't allow us to feel our feet, discourage us from developing the spring and flexibility that cushion the torso, so that we walk heavily, without feeling the quality of the ground or using the complex muscles and flexible joints of the feet, and without shifting our weight completely from one leg to the other. Our torso reacts as though its shock absorbers were gone: with tension, holding, and stress. *If you can bring the spring back into your walk, your torso will relax.* Here's a step-by-step process for learning how to do that. Like the sitting exercise described earlier, this step-by-step training process can be found in my video or DVD program, *Reduce Your Chronic Pain.*

2. *Transfer your weight from side to side.* The first step to walking more effortlessly is to learn how to shift your weight from one leg to the other actively. Start by standing with your feet slightly farther apart than your hips. Now rock slowly to the left to shift all your weight onto your left leg. *Do not bend sideways at the hip or waist.* Instead, keep your torso straight and let its entire weight shift onto your left leg. Now rock to the right, letting your entire weight shift onto the right leg. You are shifting from one leg to the other without involving your torso. Rock back and forth like this several times. Do this slowly. Feel yourself relaxing into the weight of your left leg when you shift to the left, then relaxing into the weight of the right leg when you shift to the right. When you walk correctly, in a way that reduces muscular tension, you will feel this *full shifting of weight from one foot to the other.*

3. *Push through the supporting leg to activate the gravity reflex.* Continue rocking gently and slowly from side to side, but now add a new element: as you shift your weight onto the right leg, push down into the ground with your right foot. You are pushing down

in order to drive your body up. You will feel your body becoming taller and lighter, and your left heel will tend to come off the floor. Now shift your weight onto your left leg, pushing down into the ground with your left foot. Again, you will feel your body lengthening and becoming lighter as you become taller and as your right heel comes off the floor. Now rock back and forth, transferring your weight from the right to the left and then back to the right, pushing down into the ground with the leg that is carrying the weight. You will feel not only taller and lighter but also springier. You are activating the *gravity reflex*, a reflex that helps your body to move with greater ease. Utilizing this reflex is indispensable to walking comfortably. It also makes you look and feel youthful.

To see a good example of the gravity reflex at work, look at a cat sitting up. Sitting cats have a tall, regal appearance. They use the gravity reflex: they push down into the ground with their front paws. This has the effect of lengthening and lifting their torsos, giving them a broad, beautiful chest and a royal regard. Cats push down through their limbs in order to rise up in their bodies. This pushing down to go up eliminates slumping while increasing ease. It also makes for powerful, graceful, fluid movement.

4. Transfer your weight diagonally. Once you have absorbed the feel of transferring your weight from leg to leg and of using the gravity reflex, you can begin to incorporate these into the movements that form the basis for walking. Put one foot slightly ahead and to the side of the other, as if you were starting to walk. Stand in this position and let your weight rest completely on the back leg and foot. Then push off through the *ball* of your back foot (you are using the gravity reflex) to put your weight on the front foot. Then push down with the front foot to shift your weight back again onto the back foot. Repeat this a number of times, shifting your weight diagonally from back to front and back again a number of times. Then reverse the position of your front and back feet and repeat the same exploration. It is this diagonal shifting of weight that forms the core of comfortable walking. When you find walking uncomfortable or tiring, chances are that *either you are failing to shift your weight properly, or you are failing to utilize the gravity reflex by pushing off through your back foot with each step, or both.*

5. *Go for a walk.* Use the principles of weight transfer and gravity reflex to take a walk. Begin by standing with one foot slightly ahead and to the side of the other. Push off from the ball of your back foot to transfer the weight to the front foot. Your back foot will come off the ground as you shift the weight onto your front foot. As your weight shifts fully onto the front foot, you can easily bring your back foot forward and place it in front and to the side of the other foot. Now push off again with the foot that is in back, using the gravity reflex to shift your weight onto the front foot and to give you a sense of spring. As you walk, you are shifting your weight fully from the back to the front leg and giving yourself a forward impetus by pushing off each time through the ball of your back foot, propelling yourself forward. You will feel a bounce in your walk, and your torso will swing rather than being held stiffly. Take a few minutes to walk this way, exploring how different your body feels. What do you notice?

RECOMMENDATIONS

The movement explorations described in this chapter are not meant to be isolated to ten, fifteen, or twenty minutes a day. You want to use them throughout the day, to become more aware of how you stand, sit, and walk, and to make these movements more efficient and effortless. When you move inefficiently, you carry excess tension in the torso, which can contribute to chronic pain anywhere in the body. These explorations of standing, sitting, and walking offer you ways to reduce tension in the torso and leave your muscles more relaxed. They teach you how to use your legs and feet more actively for support. Once you incorporate these approaches into your daily awareness and body use, you will dramatically improve your sense of well-being and reduce your pain. By following the suggestions given here on a daily basis for a few weeks, and using the daily log at the end of this chapter to record your progress, you will become far more sensitized to the relative levels of tension in your body and to how to reduce them. You will feel freer, lighter, and more at ease in your body, more alive. You are learning how to reduce pain—not through medication, manipulation, or strenuous and boring exercise but through deep and easy breathing, combined with an awareness of how to move in a way that eliminates needless muscular tension and stress.

If, after following the suggestions made in this book, you feel you would benefit from more training in alignment, you can pursue this by contacting either my Web site or practitioners of the Alexander Technique or Aston Patterning (see below).

FURTHER READING

Deborah Caplan, *Back Trouble* (Gainesville, FL: Triad, 1987). A solid, nuts-and-bolts approach to the Alexander Technique with lots of practical exercises, written by a former student of F. M. Alexander.

PRACTITIONERS

Alignment training is a specialty of certain kinds of movement therapists. Recommended therapies include the Alexander Technique and Aston Patterning. For information on practitioners of the Alexander Technique in your area, contact the American Society for the Alexander Technique at 1 (800) 473-0620 or www.amsat.ws. For information on practitioners of Aston Patterning, contact 1 (775) 831-8228 or www.astonenterprises.com.

Daily Alignment Exercise Log

1. Improve your alignment when standing:

Today, _____ I practiced/ _____ I did not practice:

(a) __ unlocking my knees while standing

(b) __ balancing on my feet so that my weight is neither in my heels nor in the balls of my feet, but midway between

(c) __ balancing on my feet so that my weight is distributed more on the outside of my feet than on the inside

(d) __ aligning my feet so that they point forward and are approximately hip width apart

(e) __ feeling the weight of my body distributed evenly between both legs

(f) __ feeling grounded, by growing roots and letting the earth support me.

Of the above exercises, the ones I found most useful were:

_____

2. Improve your alignment when sitting:

Today, _____ I practiced bending and going from sitting to standing/_____ did not practice bending and going from sitting to standing.

When I go from sitting to standing without thinking about it, I notice that I usually:

(a) __ hold my breath

(b) __ feel tension, effort or pain in my neck, back, hips, shoulders, etc.

(c) __ bend from the waist instead of the hip joints

(d) __ bring my knees in toward each other.

When I follow the suggestions for bending, sitting, and standing, I am able to:

(a) __ breathe in deeply when I get up from a chair

(b) __ bend from the hip joints

(c) __ let my legs instead of my torso do the work.

When I follow the instructions for bending, sitting, and standing, I find that I:

(a) __ feel more relaxed

(b) __ feel less pain

(c) __ don't notice any difference.

3. Improve your alignment when walking:

Today, ____I practiced/____did not practice the walking exercises, including:

(a) __ transferring my weight from side to side and forward and backward

(b) __ activating the gravity reflex

(c) __ applying these principles to walking.

I found that paying attention to the suggestions for walking:

(a) __ heightened my awareness of habits of walking that contribute to my pain

(b) __ made walking a little easier

(c) __ enabled me to walk without tiring as easily as usual

(d) __ felt more springy and youthful

(e) __ none of the above.

8

MINIMIZING EFFORT: A VITAL PRINCIPLE OF HEALTH

Chronic physical tension plays a central role in the etiology of chronic pain. Whatever the original source of this tension—whether mental, emotional, or physical—and whether the onset is gradual or sudden, a key element in reducing or eliminating that pain is to reduce the tension in the body. Breathing and alignment work reduce tension and can have a ripple effect that reduces pain immediately.

This chapter approaches a third way of reducing the physiological tension that underlies pain by working directly with feedback from the muscles to release subliminal muscular stress. The result: in addition to reducing your pain levels, you will find that your body will feel softer, more fluid and graceful, and younger. This body change will also trigger mental and emotional insights that will help you further manage and alleviate chronic pain.

Because people in chronic pain tend to use too much effort, reducing pain involves using less effort and working more intelligently in all your movements. That means applying minimum effort to achieve maximum results. Patricia's story sheds light on this effortless method.

PATRICIA: EXPLORING EASE IN PLACE OF EFFORT

Six weeks after she started suffering from low back pain, Patricia made an appointment with me. The onset of her back pain had occurred a day after a rather exhausting weekend during which she had entertained a number of friends at her country home. She had suffered short bouts of pain prior to this time but had not suffered from chronic pain for a number of years, since her back had bothered her for months after her father had died. Recently, Patricia had visited a chiropractor, whose manipulations had not helped her current problem. She was also in physical therapy, which she felt was helping a little, but slowly. An energetic fifty-six-year-old, Patricia found her pain distressing, and she worried that it might be the first sign of problems she associated with aging.

Observing Patricia, I saw that her back was quite swayed, so we explored how the way she sat and stood could improve her alignment. She began to feel more comfortable. Then I had Patricia lie down and show me some of the exercises she was performing in her physical therapy program. The main exercise Patricia showed me was a version of what is often called a pelvic tilt, a standard exercise for the low back. To do a pelvic tilt, you lie on your back with your knees bent and press your back against the floor. This lengthens the back muscles. In principle, the pelvic tilt can reduce chronic low back pain. In practice, however, patients rarely receive adequate instruction in how to work with this exercise, as with other exercises that could help reduce pain. Virtually every client who comes into my office and shows me his or her version of a pelvic tilt performs it in a way that at worst aggravates pain and, at best, helps it only marginally. They use too much effort, and that effort creates tension rather than release in the back. This was the case with Patricia.

As soon as Patricia lay on her back, bent her knees, and pressed her low back against the floor, I noticed that she stopped breathing. If you remember what happens when you stop breathing, you will realize that Patricia must have done the pelvic tilt in a way that tightened the muscles throughout her torso, increasing rather than reducing the torso's tension. How could this help her back? Clearly, since pain results from excess tension, what she was doing could hardly be beneficial.

I asked Patricia if she could find a way to press her back against the floor while breathing consistently. She quickly discovered that she could in fact breathe and that when she did this, she had a greater range of motion in her torso, the movement felt easier, and her back felt better. She realized that she had unwittingly been working too hard and learned how to use less effort and work more intelligently.

As we continued to explore the exercise, I made some further suggestions to Patricia to help her discover how to reduce her effort even more. Each time Patricia performed the pelvic tilt (and you will explore how to perform this movement pattern yourself in the next chapter), I asked her to repeat the movement *more gently, slowly, softly, and sensuously.* Instead of doing a typical back exercise mechanically, she was finding out how to make it a delicious, organic, sensuous experience of pleasurable movement. Since release reduces tension and release is relaxing and pleasurable, she was learning how to move with a sense of ease and pleasure. If she could perform the movement in a way that was pleasant and easy, she would automatically eliminate her neuromuscular stress. Patricia began to enjoy herself!

I asked Patricia to notice whether she could at any point in the exercise feel tension in her shoulders, neck, or abdomen. If she did, she was to see if she could inhibit those sensations of tension and move more easily. Just as in the alignment awareness exercises in chapter 7, we were following the principle that the more efficiently the body moves, the less stress you will feel in your torso and the less pain you will experience.

Patricia had never explored how she could take a simple movement and make it easier and easier. She was surprised to find that she habitually used more effort than she needed, making the exercise harder and less pleasurable than it could be and reducing the benefit to her body. Most of us are like Patricia in this regard. Have you ever noticed yourself gripping the steering wheel while you are driving? If so, you were in a state of tension and were unconsciously applying too much effort for the task at hand, which requires only a light touch. In fact, the lighter your touch on the steering wheel, the more likely you are to respond quickly and efficiently to the demands of the road. You need to minimize the effort.

When you learn to use just the right amount of effort and no more than that, you tune in to your body, and use its feedback continually to reduce the effort you bring to a task. You can see this principle at work in great athletes, whose power and beauty of movement rest on the fact that they are so keenly present to their bodies that they are able to maintain freedom of movement and a sense of grace and ease even in the most strenuous athletic performance. They minimize the effort to maximize the result.

As Patricia observed what was happening in varioius parts of her body, she discovered that her neck was especially likely to tense up when she performed the pelvic tilt. She also discovered that if she eliminated this tensing reaction, her body moved more easily. The habits we bring into exercise reflect our everyday habits. Since Patricia was tensing her neck while doing the pelvic tilt, she was undoubtedly also tensing her neck during a lot of daily activities. I therefore asked her to do two things before our next appointment. First, she was to continue to do the pelvic tilt, focusing on making the movement as gentle, smooth, soft, and effortless as possible and paying special attention to relaxing the muscles of her neck. Second, I asked her to tune in to what was happening with her neck during the day and to notice and try to release any tension there. I explained to Patricia that tension in the neck radiates down into the low back and frequently causes pain there. Even though her neck was far away from the site of her pain, it might be the real culprit in her discomfort.

Patricia came back two weeks later feeling almost well and bursting with realizations. Focusing on doing exercises in a way in which she consistently tried to make her movements softer, easier, slower, and gentler had made a big difference in her low back pain. It had also made her more aware of her habitual tension reactions. For instance, she had discovered that she frequently tensed her neck and shoulders when she was under pressure. By recognizing this and letting go of the tension repeatedly throughout the day, she felt better. Her back bothered her less, and she felt less drained.

Patricia's realizations about her body habits also had another effect: she began to see that her life was constantly focused on accomplishing tasks and making things perfect for people around her. She was always on the go, always in a state of low-grade anxiety. No wonder she continually tensed her neck!

Patricia remembered that when she was a child, her mother had frequently put on fabulous parties that had been preceded by hours or days of frantic preparations. She mused over how much her mother must have needed approval and how unpleasant she had made her own life in the process. Patricia saw that she had herself taken on some of her mother's perfectionist habits and began taking the pressure off herself. She began to learn to go at a pace that seemed more comfortable and reduced the stress in her life. Exuberantly, Patricia announced that the rewards were already coming back to her in spades. Not only was she feeling less driven, but friends and family also found it much easier to approach her. They began openly to express their appreciation for all she was doing for them, which gave her the feeling of appreciation for which she was striving. By reducing her effort, Patricia both gave and received more of what she really wanted. She walked out of my office free of pain and glowing.

Patricia's back has not bothered her since. Through bodywork, she became aware of unconscious tensions in her body and learned how to release them. This process led in turn to realizations about her own psychological defenses that helped her change her lifestyle, which improved her health. She reduced the stress level in her life, becoming gentler and kinder to herself and more receptive and open to others.

The realizations that led to the softening in Patricia's life were all triggered by her awareness of the tensions she was carrying in her body and her attempts to reduce the muscular effort and tension she felt. A simple technique for enhancing awareness of excess muscular tension—the pelvic tilt done with a focus on reducing effort and increasing ease—radiated out into fundamental life changes. Whenever Patricia got off track and reverted to her old stressful, perfectionist habits, the tensions in her body reminded her that she was drifting back into a pattern of driving herself. She used bodily feedback to keep herself on track.

"NO PAIN, NO GAIN" IS *NOT* TRUE

You can work with your muscles as Patricia did, to minimize the effort and maximize the results. But there's a difference between healing from chronic pain by emphasizing muscle strength and healing by emphasizing muscle release.

Releasing excess muscle tension involves relating to your body in a way that seems very different from the muscle strengthening of many physical therapy regimens. To learn to release muscle tension, you must focus on increasing the sensations that correspond to that release: feelings of deep relaxation, of softness, ease, fluidity, and pleasure. All the work explored in previous chapters—on breathing, alignment, and now on reducing effort—has as its goal the relaxation and enhanced flow of the body. It is certainly true that our muscles must be strong enough to support us, and some cases of chronic pain involve individual muscles that are excessively weak. However, to function efficiently, strong muscles must also be *tension-free*. A strong muscle is not a tense or hard muscle. Optimally functioning muscles are pliable and soft. Softness, or lack of tension, is perfectly compatible with strength and is essential to the effective use of muscle strength. The softness of muscles—which is different from flaccidity—is an indication of their aliveness, their availability for use in movement.

Unfortunately, muscle strengthening can be taught in a way that contributes to increasing muscle tension and rigidity rather than strength. Sometimes patients in exercise programs are told that they should push through their pain or try harder. We do need to challenge our limits, but the directive to push through pain can also have negative consequences that increase rather than decrease pain.

I once worked with an older woman who complained of extremely limited mobility in her neck, shoulders, and arms. She had been under the supervision of a physical therapist, who pushed her to work harder and harder to strengthen her upper body. When this woman worked with weights at the gym, she unwittingly gripped with her neck and shoulder muscles in every exercise. Rather than strengthening her muscles, this gripping made them tighter and tighter and less and less flexible. Her body was wound tight. She had to learn to unwind in order to regain her mobility, to reduce the effort she applied to tasks. She was already working too hard! When she learned to focus on reducing the effort she brought to tasks, her mobility improved. The key for her was to stop pushing through the pain and to stop trying harder.

Even when personal trainers or therapists don't tell you to push through pain, they may simply give you a series of exercises to perform a set number of times a day, *without paying much attention to whether or not you bring undue tension into doing the exercises*. This is what happened to Patricia. Like many patients on exercise routines, she focused on getting through exercises as quickly as possible each day, without attending to the process or feeling tone of the exercises. When we exercise, it is tempting to think that if we just do ten or twelve repetitions of our exercises each day, we will get their full benefit. If we don't enjoy the exercises, we speed through them as quickly as possible. This approach is counterproductive to reducing chronic pain and totally incompatible with learning how to reduce muscle tension. Muscle release work eliminates pain by learning how, *through slow, soft movement and attention to the body's feedback*, to make any motion more efficiently and to move more easily.

If you do not address your tension habits prior to doing muscle strengthening, you may work too hard and with inappropriate muscles. You may become discouraged because you feel pain after doing your exercises or find only limited improvement despite much hard work. Training in muscle release must *precede* training in muscle strengthening. If you first learn to release excess tension from your body, you can approach muscle-strengthening exercises without fear of further injury. By integrating the principles for minimizing effort into even the most strenuous exercises, you will enhance the positive effect of those exercises.

THE LEGACY OF MOSHE FELDENKRAIS

I learned about the critical importance of minimizing effort in order to maximize results partly through the Alexander Technique but particularly through studying Moshe Feldenkrais's system of Awareness Through Movement. Feldenkrais was a renowned master of the body who developed a unique method of healing and traveled throughout the Western world teaching it. Born in Ukraine in 1904, Feldenkrais left his home and family at the age of fourteen to emigrate to Palestine. In 1928, he moved to Paris to pursue studies in physics, mathematics, and engineering; he received his doctorate from the Sorbonne and became the principal assistant of Frédéric Joliot-Curie, who discovered induced radiation and won the 1935 Nobel Prize in Chemistry. During his time in Paris, Feldenkrais also became one of the first Europeans ever to earn a black belt in judo.

When the Nazis occupied France in 1940, Feldenkrais fled to England and worked for the British Admiralty, helping to develop sonar and other means of submarine detection. A bus accident aggravated an old knee injury, and doctors told Feldenkrais he might never walk again, even with surgery. In pursuit of a better solution than the doctors were able to offer, Feldenkrais studied everything then known about health and healing—anatomy, physiology, exercise, movement therapy, acupuncture, psychology, yoga, hypnosis, and spiritual practices. Through months of careful, minimal movements combined with close self-observation, he was able to regain the functioning of his bad knee to such an extent that he was able not only to walk but even to resume judo.

Continuing in his profession, Feldenkrais also began to work with friends and colleagues one at a time to deepen his understanding of how to facilitate healing. He felt the key to healing was to become more aware of what you were doing and that the main impediment to healing, as well as a primary cause of pain, was excess effort.

In 1950, Feldenkrais returned to Israel to become the first director of the electronics department of the Israel Defense Forces. Shortly after, he was asked to work with Israel's first prime minister, David Ben-Gurion, who suffered from severe chronic back pain, as well as other serious illnesses. His health improved so dramatically as a result of working with Feldenkrais that Feldenkrais found himself launched into fame. Accepting the challenge to teach his approach to health and healing, he left behind his engineering career and taught in Israel, Europe, and, beginning in 1971, in the United States, training large groups of practitioners in his method. He died peacefully in 1984 at the age of eighty.

Feldenkrais never systematized his work, although he wrote numerous fascinating books, because he wanted his students to discover for themselves what worked rather than taking it from him. From my own work exploring Feldenkrais's approach to movement, therefore, I have culled a number of principles that can help you reduce the effort of your own body and improve your ease. Because Feldenkrais nowhere stated these principles explicitly, I cannot say that either he or contemporary practitioners of his work would accept them, but they represent my own development of an approach to self-healing nourished by my studies of Feldenkrais.

SEVEN PRINCIPLES FOR RELEASING MUSCLE TENSION

Achieving your goal of muscle release—of working less hard and applying a minimum effort to achieving a maximum result—involves adopting seven key principles that expand upon your work with breathing and alignment. The exercises in chapter 9 assume familiarity with the following principles. It will be worth your while to study and understand these principles before exploring the exercises.

1. Feel your body. The first principle is to practice feeling your body. You already encountered this principle when you learned how to observe and accept the sensation of your breath as a means to bodily relaxation. Now you will expand your focus systematically to include nonjudgmental observation and acceptance of your body as a whole.

Tension corresponds to a decrease in sensation. The more tension you carry, the more effort you bring into your activities and the less easily you feel your body. You can reduce the tension and pain in your body and increase your sense of ease simply by heightening your sensitivity to your body's sensations, a process that automatically creates deep bodily relaxation. The first of the exercises in chapter 9 is a body scan that teaches you how to become more present to your body's sensations.

It is easy to demonstrate how increasing body awareness and sensitivity promotes relaxation. Take one hand and place it gently on your thigh. Let your fingers and palm be loose. Now become aware of the sensation of your hand. What does it feel like? However it feels is fine. There is no right or wrong, just sensation. Appreciate how your hand feels. Where exactly does your palm touch your thigh? What about your thumb? Your fingers? Now trace in your mind the contours of your hand. Trace from the base of the thumb, all the way around your thumb and each finger, to the wrist on the other side of your hand. Now imagine that your entire hand is sinking deeper and deeper into your thigh. Let it sink in. Imagine that your hand is melting. In your imagination let your palm, thumb, and fingers melt and spread into your thigh.

You have been bringing awareness to your hand. How does it feel? Do you feel it more clearly than before? Has the sensation changed? Does it feel tingly? Larger? Warmer? How does it compare to the feeling of your other hand, the hand to which you haven't been paying attention? Does the hand on which you are focusing feel bigger? More detailed? More alive? Softer? Sensations such as these correspond to deeper relaxation. By bringing your awareness to the sensation of your hand, you enhance muscle relaxation, along with the flow of blood and nerve impulses.

Your body is with you all the time. At any given time, however, you can feel it more or less clearly. The more clearly you feel it, without reacting to any sensations but just accepting them nonjudgmentally, the more relaxed it becomes and the more easily it moves. All the exercises in the next chapter reduce pain by deepening your awareness of body sensation.

When we are in pain, we may not want to feel our bodies. After all, they hurt! We take painkillers for the hurt, and painkillers dull our sensations. It is even possible, when we begin to explore the sensations of our body, that we may at first experience an increase of pain, as we are no longer blocking what is there. Nonetheless, nonjudgmental awareness of our sensations, even our sensations of pain, will tend to reduce pain *if we remain neutral and accepting of our sensations and let the body feel whatever it feels.* Nonjudgmental awareness encourages relaxation and promotes healing. Pain tends to dissipate if we don't react to it. If we react to it, it increases. When we react—when we anticipate, worry about, or are angry at our pain—we tense up. That tension causes further pain. So remember: observe how your body feels with total acceptance and curiosity. It will reward you by beginning to feel better.

As Patricia's story reminds us, feeling your body nonjudgmentally reduces chronic pain for other reasons. As you learn to be more in touch with your body from moment to moment and day to day, you become more sensitive to when and how your body tenses. Unconscious tension patterns become conscious. The good news is that while what is unconscious controls you, what becomes conscious can be controlled. By improving your awareness of your bodily tensions, you will improve your ability to release your muscle contractions and move more freely.

2. Imagine softness. As you discovered in exploring breathing, the softer you feel, the better you feel. This is because softness corresponds to a reduction of effort, and the golden rule of pain-free movement is that *less is more.* You should therefore try to reduce the effort involved in making any movement. How can you reduce effort? *The subjective sensation that corresponds to a reduction of effort is the sensation of softness.* When I worked with Patricia to reduce the effort she was bringing into doing the pelvic tilt, I repeatedly asked her to see if she could make the movement *gentler and softer*. The softer your body feels, the less tension it contains and the more freely it moves. If you sit at a computer and focus on letting your fingers feel softer and looser as they move over the keyboard, you will find yourself typing with greater ease and less effort. If you imagine that your lips, cheeks, eyes, and forehead are soft, you will eliminate tension lines from your face and worry from your mind. You will also focus more easily. If you imagine that your feet are soft and pliable as you walk, your walking will become more fluid.

In a television interview, golfing champion Tiger Woods described how he had learned to hit golf balls with ever-increasing accuracy and power. His trainer had attached a sensitive beeper to the handle of his golf club. The beeper would go off whenever Tiger gripped the club with more than a minimal amount of effort. It took Tiger time to develop the finesse and softness of touch that would keep the beeper from going off, but as he developed that soft touch, his control over his swing improved.

Tension corresponds to hardness and relaxation to softness. Make your movements softer, and you will reduce your effort and pain, while increasing the efficiency of your movements.

3. *Move slowly*. By exploring how to make a movement slowly, gently, and softly, you actually enhance your ability to move more easily and swiftly in the long run. When taking dancing lessons, you learn complex steps, and all the grace and control they require, by going through the moves slowly at first in order to master them. The process is similar when working with releasing tension patterns in your body. However, instead of learning a new movement (for example, the cha-cha), you take a habitual movement—for example, sitting up—and very slowly explore how to do it with less effort and a subtler touch. Once you have done this a number of times, you will have programmed easier movement into your body, and you will be able to make the same movement with more grace, less effort, and more speed than when you started.

Any imbalances and tensions in the body show up when we slow down our movements. I used to have balance problems. My friends sometimes called me a klutz. All that changed after I worked with slowing down my movements to gain greater control over them. For example, I worked with walking very slowly and deliberately. The more slowly I moved, the more my body was compelled to learn balance. Today, my walk is fluid and controlled and my muscles are highly responsive.

4. Start small. When you are trying to explore and release excess tension in your body, you learn more if you move slowly and start with small movements. One of the exercises in the next chapter guides you into releasing tension by making very small movements in exploring a familiar behavior pattern: rolling over. Another shows you how to release neck, back, pelvic, and overall body tension through slow, small movements. Making small, conscious movements requires you to develop a great deal of sensitivity in your body. This sensitivity corresponds to enhanced sensation and motor control. The smaller and slower you initially make your movements, the more sensitivity you develop and the greater the opportunity your muscles have to relax and regain their full range of motion and motor control.

Keeping things small requires patience. It also goes against the common assumption that stretching tight muscles as far as they can go leads to greater range and ease of motion. You will find that by starting small as well as slow, and then gradually increasing the range of your movements, you will release more tension. You will also eventually have a greater range of motion than if you started out with larger, more forceful motions.

5. Scan and release throughout your whole body. The more efficiently your body works, the fewer muscles tighten up. You discovered this principle when you explored sitting and standing. You may have noticed that before you learned to move efficiently from sitting to standing, standing up from a chair seemed to require tightening in the muscles of your thighs, abdomen, back, shoulders, and perhaps even neck. Once you learned how to stand up from a chair more efficiently, your leg muscles did most of the work, while your abdomen, back, shoulders, and neck were less involved.

As Patricia did in performing the pelvic tilt, you can vastly improve your ease of movement by learning to observe and release the tendency to tighten all the major muscle groups in your body. Each time you do an exercise, focus on reducing your overall body tension. Do the movement slowly, scan your entire body, and notice what muscles are tightening. Do you stop breathing? Do your shoulders or neck tighten up? Does your jaw tighten? What about your abdomen? You may be surprised to find how many muscles get involved in the act! See if you can gently reduce the effort throughout your body. This takes attention and patience. You are learning something new. Gradually movement will become easier.

Once you have learned to scan and release tension throughout your body, you can practice this every moment of the day—when clearing off your desk, getting up from a chair or sofa, walking into a room or down the street, washing dishes, or picking up objects. It will help you become lighter, more fluid, and freer of pain.

6. *Follow the pleasure principle.* Softness, slowness, awareness, minimizing effort, focusing on appreciating sensations—all these correspond to following the pleasure principle. Soft, slow, effortless, and sensitive movement is pleasurable movement. The more pleasurable movement is, the more efficient it is. As you experiment with your body in the exercises in chapter 9, ask yourself, "How can I make this movement in a way that feels easier and more pleasurable?" If you do this, you will most likely be your own best teacher. You will also have abundant motivation to keep learning. After all, your pain reduction program will be enjoyable!

If you start feeling pain while making a movement, consider the possibility that you may be doing too much too soon. Apply the pleasure principle. Slow down, go more gently, and make the movement smaller. Then gradually increase the size and speed of movement, staying below the pain threshold.

7. *Breathe continuously and easily.* Pay attention to your breathing, and keep it flowing. This may not be easy. By monitoring your breathing, however, you will make greater progress. Remember that your breathing style reflects what is happening to a very powerful

muscle: the diaphragm. When that muscle is relaxed and your breath is regular and deep, the rest of your body is more at ease as well.

RECOMMENDATIONS

To reduce chronic pain, you must learn how to reduce muscle tension throughout your body. The key to reducing muscle tension is to learn that efficient, pain-free movement is effortless movement. You need to minimize the effort you bring to any task in order to maximize your bodily efficiency and let go of subliminal stress.

Apply the seven principles described above to the movement patterns discussed in the next chapter. These patterns are, technically speaking, not exercises. They are explorations that can change the way you move from day to day. Learning muscle release techniques is not about spending fifteen minutes a day doing something with your body and then forgetting about it. It is about learning how to change the way you use your body, so that you will move more fluidly and easily from moment to moment. That's what makes for pain reduction and healing.

FURTHER READING

Moshe Feldenkrais, *Awareness Through Movement* (New York: Harper & Row, 1972). The classic work on Feldenkrais's system of Awareness Through Movement, presented by its founder.

Moshe Feldenkrais, *The Potent Self: A Guide to Spontaneity* (New York: Harper & Row, 1985). A fascinating exploration of the relationship between freedom of movement and creativity.

9

LETTING GO OF EFFORT
TO LET GO OF PAIN

Learning to move with less effort is highly pleasurable and creates a deep sense of peace. Because doing so requires focus and attention, the four explorations described below will each help you in this process in a different way. The first will teach you to reduce your body tension through total body awareness. The second takes a simple movement pattern—rolling over—and shows you how to do it more easily than most people do. In the process of making one simple movement more effortless, you will learn how to extrapolate to other daily movements. The third exercise takes you through a typical back exercise, the pelvic tilt, and shows how to perform that exercise more pleasurably and efficiently to reduce your back pain. Again, you will be able to extrapolate concepts from this learning and apply them to other exercises. The fourth exploration shows you how to use gentle movement while standing to free blockages and tensions throughout your body.

Use the daily log at the end of this chapter to keep track of your progress in exploring the four movement patterns described in this chapter. Use this log until you have learned how to bring your awareness into daily movement to minimize your effort and maximize your results.

THE BODY SCAN

Like the breath awareness exercise, this one teaches you to relax deeply by absorbing the sensations of your body in a nonjudgmental, accepting manner. I first discovered the power of nonjudgmental observation and acceptance of my body while I was lying in bed, full of self-pity because I was feeling poorly. My left knee was killing me! My usual reaction was simply to feel miserable about it, to obsess about the pain, and possibly to take a painkiller. This particular night, however, something compelled me to try a different tack. I decided that rather than being upset or agitated about the pain, I would simply observe it, with the same detachment that one might feel when watching the wind blow through trees or looking at cells under a microscope. I observed my pain in an open, curious, but emotionally neutral manner, noticing that when I did this, the pain didn't seem to affect me as much.

After a few minutes, something interesting happened. The pain dissipated. Then it disappeared altogether. This was intriguing, because usually when I paid attention to my pain, it either stayed constant or increased. Apparently, the way I was observing it now had a different impact. The combination of interest and detachment, so different from the worry and fear I usually brought to my awareness of pain, had triggered a relaxation response. Once my body got the message that it could feel however it wanted to, it simply relaxed, and my pain went away.

In the years that followed, I explored the principle of releasing muscle tension through observing and accepting sensations thousands of times. Every night before I went to sleep, I would scan my entire body in the way described in the exercise below. By the end of the body scan, I was usually on the edge of a deep and peaceful sleep. This had an unexpectedly positive consequence. Like many people in chronic pain, I was used to waking up stiff and sore in the morning. Over a number of months, the soreness and stiffness completely disappeared. By focusing on deep relaxation every evening, I trained my body out of a chronic unconscious tension pattern that it had adopted while I was asleep.

People commonly tense their muscles during sleep. Some clench their jaw, others their neck or shoulders, hands, or feet. In the depths of sleep, when our conscious minds no longer exert control, primitive emotions of fear and anger can come up and affect our bodies. Consciously releasing tension before sleep can retrain this destructive process.

Use the body scan below at any time of day or night, sitting or lying down. Read the exercise into a tape or order a copy of the body scan cassette or CD through my Web site, or by using the order form at the end of the book.

At first, it may take you ten or fifteen minutes to experience this exercise thoroughly. Once you have absorbed all it has to teach you, you will be able to scan your entire body in just a few moments.

1. *Take a moment to focus inward without distractions.* Find a quiet place. Lie down on your back on a firm surface or sit in a chair, relaxed but erect, feet flat on the floor and spine straight, feeling the support of your sitz bones beneath you and with your head poised nicely over your spine. Close your eyes to focus your attention more clearly on your sensations. Can you feel your breathing?

Calm yourself by following your breath. Rest your attention on the feeling of your breath moving into and out of your body until you feel quiet and focused. Now you are ready to observe your body sensations.

2. *Appreciate the sensations of your right leg.* Become aware of the sensation of your right foot, including the heel, the ball, the toes, and the top. If you cannot feel your foot clearly, squeeze and release your toes a few times. Observe how your foot feels, and appreciate that. How it feels is exactly as it should feel. Then expand your awareness to include your right calf. When you feel both your right foot and calf clearly, include your right thigh in your awareness.

Enjoy picking up the information your body sends you. Avoid judgment. Notice any temptation you may have to label a sensation as bad or worrisome. If you feel pain or discomfort, allow yourself to register it without comment. This will allow the sensation to pass through and dissipate.

3. *Appreciate the sensations of your left leg.* Shift your attention to your left foot, absorbing how it feels. Then include the calf in your awareness. Once you feel the foot and calf clearly, become aware of the thigh as well. What do you notice? Observe, appreciate, and accept, allowing your left leg to feel exactly as it feels.

4. *Appreciate the sensations of both your right and left legs.* Can you feel both legs simultaneously? You are gradually including more and more of your body in your awareness. What does it feel like? Does your body feel different? How? Register any changes without judgment.

5. *Appreciate the sensations of your pelvis and abdomen.* Shift your attention to your pelvic area. Become aware of the sensation of your right buttock, then your left buttock. What do they feel like? Let the sensations sink in. Then become aware of your abdomen, so that you are now feeling your entire lower torso. Take your time. Then include in your awareness both your right and left legs and your pelvis and abdomen.

6. *Appreciate the sensations of your entire torso.* Shift your attention to your entire torso. Become aware of the feeling of the front of your torso, including your ribs and your chest, both to the left and to the right. What does your torso feel like? What about the back of your torso: your ribs in back and your shoulders? Can you feel both the front and back of your torso simultaneously? Become aware of the feeling of your neck, on the right, on the left, in front, and in back. Now become aware of the feeling of your torso along with your legs. Absorb the sensations.

7. *Appreciate the sensations of your arms.* Bring your awareness to the feeling of your right arm, from the shoulder to the elbow, the elbow to the wrist, and the wrist to the tips of your fingers. Now feel your whole right arm. Absorb what it feels like. Then do the same thing with your left arm, moving from the shoulder to the elbow, the elbow to the wrist, the wrist to the fingertips, and then absorbing the feeling of the whole arm. Now feel both arms together. Now feel your arms, your torso, and your legs simultaneously. How do you feel?

8. *Appreciate the sensations of your head.* Become aware of the feeling of the front of your face. Take time to include your lips, your

cheeks, the area under your eyes, and your forehead. Now feel the sides of your head, around your ears, then the back of your head. Now feel the front, sides, and back of your head simultaneously. What does this feel like?

9. *Appreciate the sensations of your entire body.* Become aware of your entire body, including the feet, legs, torso, arms, hands, and head. Notice and appreciate what this feels like. What has changed? How does your body feel different? Is it lighter? Heavier? More tingly? Can you feel more of yourself more clearly? Do you feel more comfortable? Often, pain will go away just as a result of your becoming more present to your body.

10. *Now that you have finished the exercise,* see if you can begin to practice simple body awareness throughout the day. It will automatically reduce tension and pain.

ROLL OVER; MOVE LIKE A BABY

Every morning when we get out of bed, we roll over. Every time we do this, we use our bodies either efficiently or inefficiently. When we use them efficiently, our movement feels relatively effortless. When we use them inefficiently, the movement involves effort—feelings of tension, strain, or stress in the neck, shoulders, back or abdomen, and hips. Chances are, you have never paid attention to how much effort you use in rolling over to get out of bed or off a sofa or up from the floor. You just assume that the effort that you expend is the effort you have to expend. But this is far from the truth.

Ninety percent of the people I work with roll over inefficiently to get out of bed and unconsciously create pain in their bodies. Observing and imitating how a baby rolls over helps us to see how to reduce our effort and increase efficiency. This movement pattern teaches you how to roll over using your body efficiently, like a baby. (For an audiovisual presentation, see my video or DVD *Reduce Your Chronic Pain.*)

1. *Self-observation.* Lie down on the floor or on a firm surface, and then roll onto your side. First roll to the left a few times, then to

the right. What muscles are working? Do you feel tension in your neck, shoulders, abdomen, back, legs, or arms? Are you breathing easily, or do you hold your breath or breathe with difficulty? Make note of what you observe before exploring how to roll over more easily.

2. *Use your legs and hips to initiate rolling, eliminating tension elsewhere.* Lie down again on your back, bend your left leg, and put your left foot on the floor. Find a place where it feels as though your left leg is most balanced or takes the least effort to hold it up. Your right leg should be fully extended. Now press down into the floor with your left foot. As you do this, check to see that your left knee is over your foot and is pointed up, as opposed to going from side to side. You will feel your left hip rising slightly as you press down with your left foot. You will also feel your body weight shifting toward your right pelvis. Repeat this movement a number of times, pressing down on your left foot and feeling your body shift over toward the right. As you do this, notice the following:

    a. Is your right leg (your extended leg) stiff? Can you relax it more?

    b. Are you breathing easily, without interruption, as you make the movement?

    c. Can you relax your shoulders, neck, torso, and abdomen? Can you feel your whole body while you are pressing your foot into the floor? Can you eliminate all effort except for the effort made by your left foot pressing into the floor? Can the rest of your body be like a rag doll?

    d. Can you make the movement of your left leg and hip slower, softer, smaller, and smoother? How slow? How soft? How small? How smooth? What does it feel like when you make the motion more subtle? What are you learning?

    e. Experiment with different foot positions for your left foot, moving it closer to and further from your buttocks. Find the place from which it is easiest to move your hip.

Repeat the movement of your left leg, gradually increasing the speed and range of movement, until it feels quite easy and broad. Can you feel how, as your left foot presses down, your left hip extends upward and your back arches, while your shoulders stay on the ground? You are giving yourself a pleasant stretch! Now repeat the entire process with your right leg bent and your left leg straight on the floor. Start slow, small, and soft, relaxing your body and breathing easily. Then gradually increase the range and speed of movement. Take all the time you need. Can you feel how your body begins to roll to the left as you press down with the right foot?

3. *Expand the rolling motion to roll over fully.* Now continue to lie flat on the floor, but bend your legs so that both feet are on the floor and your legs feel comfortably balanced.

a. Let both legs drop comfortably to the *right* and rest there for a moment, allowing your entire body to relax into this position. (If your legs feel a strain, put some pillows under them, to the right side of your body. This will break the fall of your legs at a place where you get some stretch but are still comfortable.) Then bring your legs back to the center. (You will find it easier to do this if you inhale as you bring your legs back to the upright position. Inhaling inhibits the tendency to use unnecessary tension.)

Repeat this movement a number of times, dropping your legs to the right, relaxing fully, then inhaling as you bring your legs back to center. Explore how easily you can do this. Can you breathe throughout? Notice if you feel any tension, for example in the neck, throat, or abdomen. Can you let go of this tension and let your legs drop without any resistance? Can you bring your legs back to an upright position without clenching in your torso? Now do the same thing, this time letting your legs drop to the *left*, resting and relaxing, and then inhaling as you bring them back to center. Do this a number of times. Then let your legs fall easily and gently to the right, come back to center, fall to the left, come back to center, to the right, and so on. Breathe. Relax your entire body.

b. Let your legs drop to the right, and while you do this, press down with your left foot, in the same way as you did in No. 2 above. Can you feel your entire pelvis and lower torso rolling to the right while your shoulders stay on the floor? Repeat this movement a few times. Then make the same movement, letting your legs drop to the left and pressing down with your right foot to roll your pelvis and lower torso to the left. Repeat a number of times. See how easily you can do this. Then roll first to the right and then to the left. See how smooth, soft, and pleasurable you can make the movement.

c. Now let your legs drop to the right again, pressing down with your left foot to roll your pelvis to the right. This time let your left arm and shoulder come off the floor as well and roll your upper torso to the right. You will end up on your side with your face looking to the right. Repeat this motion a number of times, allowing your shoulder and upper torso to follow the movement of your pelvis with minimum effort. You have rolled over effortlessly! Repeat the same maneuver, letting your legs drop to the left as you press down with your right foot, rolling your pelvis to the left, and letting your right arm and shoulder and upper torso follow the movement of your pelvis.

d. Compare how you are rolling over now with the way you started. What has changed? Has rolling become easier for you? You have learned how to initiate rolling with the legs in a way that releases and lengthens the muscles of your entire torso while reducing effort.

e. The steps outlined above have taught you how to roll from your back onto your side, using minimum effort by initiating the movement with your legs, letting both legs fall to the side while the torso stays relaxed, and then letting your shoulder and upper torso follow your legs. Make a point of noticing how you roll over in bed or when you are on the floor. Can you improve your movement and make it more effortless? Integrate what you have learned into your daily life.

THE PELVIC TILT

Properly performed, this movement pattern is extraordinarily effective in relieving back pain and toning and stretching the muscles of the torso. Simultaneously, it teaches you how to recognize and release excess tension. It is an excellent movement to use first thing in the morning before getting out of bed, lying in bed at night, or anytime the body feels stiff and tight. Once you have learned, through practicing the pelvic tilt, how to incorporate the seven principles of freer movement described in chapter 8 into your exercises, you can use these principles to explore any type of movement lying down and to release tension throughout your entire body. (A visual presentation of this exercise can be found in my video or DVD *Reduce Your Chronic Pain.*)

1. *Find a comfortable position lying down.* Lie on your back with your hands at your sides. Bend your knees and place your feet hip width apart. Explore how close to each other and to your buttocks your feet need to be in order for your legs to feel as balanced and relaxed as possible. Put a pillow under your head if your neck needs support.

2. *Breathe and scan your body.* Spend a few moments breathing diaphragmatically, or into your belly. Feel your belly expand as you breathe in and retract as you breathe out. Let your body sink into the surface underneath you, feeling its full support. Scan your body for signs of tension. Can you let go of tension in your face, jaw, neck, shoulders, chest, abdomen, and legs? Continue to breathe in a soft, relaxed manner.

3. *Roll your pelvis forward and backward.* Gently begin to arch and then flatten your back. As you arch your back, the small of your back will move away from the floor and your pelvis will roll forward. As you flatten your back, the small of your back will press into the floor and your pelvis will roll back. Notice the motion of your pelvis. Make this motion as slow, soft, and fluid as possible. If you experience any pain, make the movement smaller, until you feel little or no pain.

Repeat this gentle, soft motion of arching and rounding your back ten or fifteen times.

4. *Notice your breathing*. Have you stopped breathing while arching and rounding your back? If so, you are working against yourself. Try to breathe regularly and deeply as you move between arching and rounding. Make relaxed breathing your top priority! Do you breathe in or out as you arch your back? Explore which one feels easier. You will discover that it is easier to breathe in as you arch your back and out as you round your back. This is because your abdomen expands when you arch and gets smaller when you round your back.

Once your breath is free and fluid, do you notice that the entire movement of arching and rounding your back seems easier?

5. *Notice what muscles are working*. What muscles tighten as you arch and flatten your back? Does your abdomen clench? What about your shoulders? Your neck? Your jaw? Your chest? Your thighs and calves? Pay close attention. Slow the movement way down if you need to, in order to see what muscles are working.

All those who do this exercise notice muscular effort in their legs as they arch and round the back. This is natural. At first, however, most people also observe tension in their abdomen and sometimes in their shoulders, chest, jaw, or neck. This tension *reduces flexibility while increasing effort*.

6. *Release tension in the torso*. While you are arching and rounding your back, see if you can consciously relax your abdomen, jaw, neck, and shoulders. You will be able to do this if you *let your legs do the work*. Press your feet into the floor to flatten your back. Then arch your back by pulling gently with your feet. (It might help to imagine that your feet are suction cups.) Let your entire body, with the exception of your legs, be like a rag doll, soft and limp. Can you feel how much easier the movement becomes?

7. *Explore the wave*. Continue to breathe out as you press down with your feet to round your back, and breathe in as you pull with your feet to arch your back. Is the movement becoming easier? Are you feeling more flexible? More relaxed? Softer? How gliding, gentle, soft, and slow can you make the motion? Is the movement becoming

larger and freer? Does it begin to feel easy and wavelike? Go into the wave. Play with the movement for a minute or longer.

8. *Rest, observe, and digest.* When you have finished exploring the movement, rest for a few moments. How does your body feel? Have you discovered that movement is easier when you breathe fully and release tension from the torso? Can you incorporate this understanding into your everyday movements? For example, after resting, see if you can roll over and stand up while breathing easily and feeling minimum tension in your shoulders, neck, jaw, and abdomen. Can you let your legs do 90 percent of the work and let your torso be relaxed? You are learning how to move efficiently and therefore with less pain.

9. *Apply your learning to everyday movement.* Use this gentle exercise to free up tension and stretch your spine on a daily basis. In addition, apply what you have learned to your everyday life. Notice, as you sit in a chair, lean forward or back, stand or walk, whether you stop breathing or whether you tighten muscles in your abdomen, shoulders, neck, or jaw. Slowly and gently explore whether you can find a way to move with less tension while breathing deeply. Be patient in your practice, and it will reward you with greater physical ease.

MOVE LIKE A CAT—WITH FLOW

I frequently teach classes on chronic pain reduction for older people in their sixties and beyond. First I show them—through movement patterns like those above—that consciously focusing on making small, slow, soft, gentle movements with the body gradually reduces muscle tension and pain. Then I show them how to apply these principles to releasing tension and pain *from any part of their bodies*. I am always astonished at how quickly people who may have suffered from pain for years respond to the simple approach described below. All this approach requires is that you learn to listen to your own feedback and use it to become more pliable within yourself.

You do not need specific exercises, and you do not need to go to an orthopedist or a physical therapist, to learn how to listen to what your body needs and to apply the seven principles for releasing muscle tension to reducing pain in any part of your body. Below, you will explore how to do this, beginning with your neck and then moving down your spine. (A visual presentation of this exercise can be found on my video or DVD.)

1. *Stand or sit in a relaxed position.* Focus on your breath and see if you can gently move into deeper diaphragmatic breathing. At the same time, scan your body for any tension in the face, neck, shoulders, arms, abdomen, back, and legs. As far as possible, release any tension you find. Throughout this exercise, continue to scan your body and to release excess tension.

2. *Explore slow, soft neck movements.* Allow your neck to drop slowly and gently to the right. Absorb the sensation. Then gently let the neck drop forward, then over to the left side. Do this as slowly as possible. Then allow the head to fall back gently, and again over to the right. Move softly and slowly, and allow for *small* rather than large movements. You are giving the neck time to relax, to use the weight of gravity to stretch itself out, and to find underutilized muscles. Do not force any movement. Let yourself be interested in the sensations of your neck. Repeat this movement a few times, continuing to focus on soft, slow, small, and gentle motions. You can continue to do this for several minutes if you like, as the movement will feel increasingly pleasurable.

Note: While you are rolling your neck to the sides and forward and back, you are *not* doing a typical "neck roll." These are usually done rapidly and without attention to absorbing the sensation of the neck. Your main goal here is not to *do* something but to *feel* your neck from the inside out, to let the neck tell you what it needs to release, open up, and feel looser.

3. *Expand the neck movements playfully.* Now let your neck find its own way to stretch out softly, gently, slowly, and playfully. Become your neck! Feel from the inside out where your neck wants to stretch itself. Experiment with letting your neck become sensuous. How does it want to move in order to feel better, to work out the kinks, even to feel really good? Continue to play with this for several minutes. You

will gain the full benefit of this exercise only if you give yourself plenty of time.

4. *Invite your shoulders into the movement.* By now your neck has been having such a good time, perhaps your shoulders want to join the fun! Feel how they want to move to free themselves up. There are no rules here. Everyone's body needs to move differently. Allow yourself to *feel like a cat.* Let your shoulders tell you how they want to stretch and move. Explore the sensations of your neck and shoulders for a minute or longer.

5. *Let your torso join in.* Perhaps your chest, rib cage, or back muscles would like to engage and stretch themselves out a bit. Let your torso begin to move, exploring what feels good. Move from the inside out. If your body feels uncomfortable anywhere, let the muscles that are uncomfortable decide how they need to move. Your body knows better than you how to fix itself. Trust in your body's ability to stretch itself out when you tune in to its needs.

6. *Continue this exploration of flow with your whole body.* Continue letting your whole body move, slowly, softly, finding the places deep inside that need stretching, that need to feel themselves. Let your entire body find its own unique way of moving and stretching. You can do this for a few minutes or for an hour. Enjoy the experience.

7. *Rest, digest, and reflect.* Rest and absorb how differently your body feels. Do you feel more alive? More energized and relaxed? You have been listening to your body's wisdom. By moving slowly and softly to begin with, you have gotten in touch with your body's sensations. Rather than manipulating yourself, you have allowed your sensations to guide you to what you need. This is the essence of spontaneous, self-regulated stretching.

8. *Stretch like a cat when you are in pain—as well as just for fun.* A daily spontaneous body stretch provides a wonderful tool for staying young, as well as for reducing chronic tension and pain. It doesn't take long—five to fifteen minutes at most—and if you like, it can be done to the accompaniment of your favorite music.

RECOMMENDATIONS

Movement that focuses on learning how to be slow, soft, gentle, and self-aware, and that explores small changes in position, is movement that teaches your body how to release subliminal tensions that contribute to aging and pain. This type of movement work increases the fluidity of your body, teaches you how to feel deep pleasure, and also helps you identify and let go of daily habits of stress.

This chapter has explored four awareness patterns that can help you to minimize your effort and maximize your results, or to move increasingly effortlessly: a body scan, rolling over, the pelvic tilt, and moving like a cat. Not only is each awareness pattern healing in itself, it also teaches you how to extrapolate the principles of healthy movement to all your daily movements. Lie on the floor or observe your daily movements, and practice becoming softer, smoother, and more effortless. Use the daily log at the end of this chapter to record your experiences. Observe the result in a reduction of your pain.

Movement awareness of this kind can be profoundly healing. If, after exploring the recommendations made here, you wish to pursue more of this type of work, you can contact my Web site for training programs or look into finding a Feldenkrais practitioner (see below).

FURTHER READING

Thomas Hanna, *Somatics* (New York: Addison-Wesley, 1988). A clear exploration of how stress creates muscle tension, along with movement patterns to release that tension, by a former student of Feldenkrais who founded a form of bodywork called Somatics.

Frank Wildman, *The Busy Person's Guide to Easier Movement* (Berkeley, Calif.: Intelligent Body Press, 2000). A concise guide to movement patterns for freeing up the body, by a teacher of Feldenkrais Awareness Through Movement.

PRACTITIONERS

Feldenkrais practitioners are among the very best movement therapists for training in how to apply minimum effort to achieve maximum results. For information on Feldenkrais practitioners in your area, contact the Feldenkrais Guild of North America in Albany, Oregon, at 1 (800) 775-2118 or www.feldenkrais.com. Excellent tapes and audio programs are also available through the Feldenkrais Movement Institute, headed by Feldenkrais practitioner and trainer Frank Wildman. The Feldenkrais Movement Institute, located in Berkeley, California, can be contacted at 1 (800) 342-3424 or www.feldenkraisinstitute.org.

Daily Movement Awareness Log

1. The body scan:
Today, _____ I practiced/ _____ I did not practice:
_____ feeling my entire body while lying down.

I noticed that when I practice whole-body awareness:
(a) __ I feel physically more relaxed
(b) __ I do not feel physically more relaxed
(c) __ sometimes I have less pain
(d) __ I do not have less pain.

2. Roll over; move like a baby:
Today, _____ I explored rolling to my side/ _____ I did not explore rolling to my side.

I noticed that:
(a) __ I found it easier to roll to my side when I followed
      the exercise
(b) __ I did not find it easier to roll to my side when
      I followed the exercise.

3. The pelvic tilt:
Today, _____ I practiced the pelvic tilt for ___ minutes/ _____ I did not practice the pelvic tilt.

I noticed that:
(a) __ the movement helped relieve tension or pain
(b) __ the movement did not help relieve tension or pain
(c) __ I felt better overall after doing the movement
(d) __ I noticed no change after doing the movement
(e) __ the movement is helping me become more aware
      of excess effort in daily activities
(f) __ the movement is not helping me become more aware
      of excess effort in daily activities.

4. Move like a Cat—with Flow

Today, _____I practiced letting go of tension through flow
for _____minutes/_____I did not practice letting go of tension
through flow.

I noticed that:

(a) __ the movement helped relieve tension or pain
(b) __ the movement did not help relieve tension or pain
(c) __ I felt better overall after doing the movement
(d) __ I noticed no change after doing the movement.

Part III

YOUR
FEELINGS

LETTING GO OF
EMOTIONAL STRESS

10

BURIED EMOTIONS FEED PAIN

The first exercise of chapter 9 was a body scan that taught you how to release tension in your body by slowly and gradually scanning your entire body while being present to your sensations without reaction. Being present to your body's sensations is inherently relaxing. If you have already practiced this body scan, you may also have noticed that focusing on feeling your *sensations* can seamlessly transition into feeling your *feelings*. Feelings are, after all, sensations.

Feeling your sensations nonjudgmentally can release tension and pain. Because feeling your sensations can lead to feeling *unacknowledged* feelings, it is possible that experiencing these previously buried feelings can also release physical pain, as the following story demonstrates.

WHEN FEELING YOUR BODY BRINGS UP EMOTIONS

A number of years ago, I was giving a class on movement awareness and muscle release and asked for someone to volunteer as a subject for the body scan. An elegant sixty-five-year-old woman named Lucia took up the challenge. I knew little about her beyond the fact that she had had a very rough time for a few months the year before, when chronic pain had confined her to a body brace and she had been hospitalized. She still suffered from pain, but it was no longer severe enough to immobilize her.

Lucia lay down on the bodywork table. I guided her through the body scan, encouraging her to release her tension by observing her body's sensations and accepting them without judgment. After a few minutes, Lucia's face began to quiver. Soon the quivering changed to tremors that passed through her body, becoming increasingly violent. Finally, unable to further restrain the flood within, Lucia began to weep. Giant waves of emotional pain washed through her body. The class participants supported her with a compassionate silence. As Lucia gave vent to her emotions, the tension and hard lines visibly ebbed from her body.

Once Lucia's tears subsided, she shared what she could grasp of her experience. She hadn't known before she lay down that she was full of emotional pain. In fact, she had felt quite contained and in control of herself, although she had recognized that she was nervous and tense. "After a few minutes connecting to the feeling of my body," she said, "I became calmer. Then some strong feelings of grief and anger welled up inside me." Those emotions felt as though they had been there a long time and were demanding acknowledgment. Feeling safe in the environment of the class, Lucia had let it all out.

Lucia recognized what the grief and anger were about. Her husband had died the previous year. A severe heart condition that had kept him housebound had made him heavily dependent on her for close to ten years before his death. Day after day, week after week, month after month, year after year, she had been the kind, dutiful wife, taking care of a man who was not only ill but also ill tempered. Trapped in a depressing, hostile environment, Lucia had felt incapable of taking space for herself. She had been full of inner pain over her own suffering in the situation and of an anger toward her husband that she felt she could not express because he was sick and dependent. She had battened down the hatches on her own feelings and had focused all her energies on getting the job done. Now, however, relieved of the burden of her husband's last years, she could afford to let go of coping. She could feel her feelings.

For years, Lucia had felt that her situation required her to ignore her feelings. She had split her mind and heart off from each other and had become increasingly out of touch with her feelings. This had inevitably put her out of touch with her body as well. The conflict between her mind and heart, her mental and emotional lives, had registered itself as an unconscious decision *not* to feel. The body scan, by encouraging a relaxation of physical tensions, gave her explicit permission to feel, and she released the iron grip she had imposed on herself.

When Lucia left the class later that day, she remarked on how much freer and lighter her body felt. She also said she was more at peace. Over the following weeks, Lucia came for a series of private sessions. Her physical pain continued to dissolve.

Feeling connects physical and emotional pain. Emotions are feelings, and feelings are sensations that reside in the body. Grief may be a pressure in the throat or a heaviness in the chest; anger, a clenching in the jaw or a tightening in the solar plexus; fear, a tightening of the gut or neck. Because feelings express themselves viscerally, if they are not released and are instead denied or controlled, the resulting tensions compromise the body's functions. Tension that is maintained rather than released creates a condition of *not* feeling. The less we feel our feelings, the more tension we carry in our bodies. The less we feel our bodies, the more pain we suffer.

Tension can be a way of avoiding or blocking feeling. Once we own our emotions fully, the tension that holds them back can let go. A male colleague of mine suffered a traumatic fall during a biking trip. He experienced severe shock along the length of one side of his body from the impact of the fall. He also cut his face deeply, almost lost one eye, and had to undergo emergency room surgery. A few days after his fall, he insisted to me that he was coping just fine. He rejected offers of assistance, saying there was no need. Six weeks later, he agreed to see me because he continued to have discomfort in his face, neck, and shoulders. Even so, as he walked in the door, he protested, "It's really nothing." For half an hour, I encouraged him to feel his body's sensations. I mobilized this process by gently touching the affected parts of his body. Finally, the tears came. This strong man began to own the feelings of vulnerability and shock he had endured as a result of his life-threatening accident. As he cried quietly, his physical pain gradually dissipated and his body relaxed.

My colleague was a man, and men aren't supposed to cry. He was also a high achiever who had grown up in a family that was emotionally unexpressive. Identified with his competency, he was always on the go, coping with the next problem. He assumed that any feelings of vulnerability should be dismissed and pushed aside as insignificant. Because he hadn't allowed himself fully to feel the physical and emotional shock of his trauma, it had stayed locked in his body. Once he allowed himself to process that shock and feel his own human vulnerability, he could feel better both physically and emotionally.

Lucia's chronic pain was of long duration, persisting over years during which she had denied her own emotional life. My colleague's pain was of shorter duration and less emotional complexity, reflecting primarily his sense that as a man and a competent achiever, he couldn't afford to be emotionally vulnerable. Both cases, however, exemplify a common problem: we may develop pain because we consciously or unconsciously reject our feelings as inappropriate. Eventually, this process puts us so much out of touch with our bodies and our feelings that it can take considerable time to reconnect to our inner reality and to allow our emotional life full expression.

As I am a body-centered therapist, one of my jobs is to help my clients get into contact with buried feelings that may be contributing to their pain. One of the ways I do this is to combine body awareness work with touch and dialogue that help clients explore how they feel in their bodies. The stories of Eileen and Bob, below, demonstrate how suppressing the right to feel creates pain and disease and how professional guidance in feeling your body can help you heal from physical pain as you become comfortable with owning your emotions.

EILEEN: LEARNING HOW TO FEEL

When Eileen first came into my office, she seemed lively, energetic, and happy. For a year and a half, however, she had been suffering from involuntary spasms and tremors, vertigo, sudden adrenaline rushes, hyperactivity, and insomnia. Her doctors had tentatively diagnosed her as having Lyme disease and put her on a prolonged course of antibiotics and antidepressants, which had given her only temporary relief. She had embarked on a quest for further assistance. By the time she came to visit me, she had seen numerous doctors, nutritionists, and homeopaths, with limited results.

The cheerful, competent demeanor of this woman who was in such great physical discomfort struck me. Despite her ailments, Eileen worked long hours as an occupational therapist and was the main support of her family. In the course of our first session, Eileen revealed that both her parents were Holocaust survivors. As a child, Eileen had participated in numerous family events that had involved watching graphic documentaries of World War II concentration camps. This was a form of therapy for her mom and dad, but for Eileen it had been traumatic. Even more challenging for Eileen was that, like many Holocaust survivors, her parents had had great difficulty either expressing or accepting any expression of emotion. It seemed to me that Eileen's cheerful, can-do demeanor might be a result of the emotional prohibitions of her childhood. Eileen confessed that she rarely cried and that she felt driven to approach life at a fast pace.

I put Eileen on a bodywork table and introduced her to the meditative breathing and the body scan exercises. When I work with a client, I also utilize palpation skills I have developed through training in craniosacral therapy, a scientifically based, very gentle manual therapy that is particularly useful in the treatment both of chronic pain and of central nervous system and endocrine disorders. (The word "craniosacral" is derived from "cranium," or head, and "sacrum," or base of the spine.) Craniosacral therapists are highly trained in the art of palpation—the ability to diagnose and treat physical problems through the use of touch—which can be an efficient technique for identifying the location of fascial and neuromuscular restrictions that might be causing chronic pain. Palpation skills are particularly important because the location of restrictions in the body is often different from the location of symptoms. Focusing only on symptoms—a sore shoulder or a low back problem—may be an inefficient way of addressing a pain problem. Skilled palpation, however, can lead you straight to the underlying cause of pain.

When I use palpation to identify areas of restriction, I sometimes put my hands over those areas to help mobilize tissue release and energize the client's awareness of these parts of the body. I also sometimes suggest that the client bring her attention to these areas, to be present to them, and to notice how they feel. In my sessions with Eileen, I also asked her to accept any sensations she felt nonjudgmentally and to share them if it felt right.

During the course of her first session, Eileen noticed that her pain became less intense. And to her surprise, the more her body relaxed, the more feelings of sadness welled up. Reflecting on how hard she had been pushing herself year after year, Eileen shed a few tears. Was it any surprise that her body had been compelled to collapse if she could never let go?

Between her first and second sessions, Eileen worked with tension release at home, utilizing the meditative breath awareness and the body scan exercises and paying attention to her breathing throughout the day. She made it a conscious goal to train her body to release some of its stress and felt she had made some improvement by the time she visited me again.

On her second visit, I drew Eileen's attention to her left hip, which palpation told me was particularly blocked. As Eileen explored the sensations in her left hip, she remarked that it felt both numb and compressed, as if something were being pressed hard against her left side. The more she brought attention gently into this area, the more it began to spasm and pain her. As she stayed with the sensations rather than judging or reacting to them, the spasms gradually worked themselves through. Eileen felt the pain receding, and the whole left side of her body lengthened and softened. She felt much better.

Why did Eileen's pain first intensify and then dissipate? If you have ever experienced frostbite in your fingers, you know that intense cold numbs your fingers. You also know that as circulation and warmth return to them, you experience pain. This pain is an indication of a return to health and normalcy. The pain first increases and then lessens as the constriction in the blood vessels relaxes. The situation is similar with chronic pain. Focusing on nonjudgmentally feeling your body stimulates constructive nerve activity and may initially cause an increase in pain, but this is generally followed by a decrease. Simply by accepting her physical sensations, Eileen triggered a healing response.

Then Eileen began to have a panic attack. The physiological relaxation she was experiencing was frightening. It felt dangerous because tension had been her way of staying alert, on guard, and defended against unknown dangers. Throughout her life, Eileen's tension had been her way of both camouflaging and controlling underlying feelings of fear that she had developed growing up as the child of Holocaust survivors. By letting go of her tension, she exposed herself to her raw fear, and this made her more anxious.

I asked Eileen to see if she could stay with her feelings of fear without reacting to them. I encouraged her to focus on her breathing, one breath at a time. This would give her a little distance from her panic and allow her to detach. Eileen struggled with this but over the next few minutes successfully faced her fear by anchoring herself in her breathing. Her panic gradually subsided. Eileen learned an important lesson during this process: while we often avoid our feelings for fear of being overwhelmed, if we can allow ourselves to experience them, even the worst feelings eventually dissipate and dissolve. When we fear being overwhelmed, we put our feelings under lock and key. They then control our behavior by requiring a rigid defense system that can create pain. When we allow ourselves to have our feelings, they lose their power, and we can let go of our rigid tensions of defense.

At the end of this session, Eileen not only felt better physically—softer, more flexible, more physically relaxed and comfortable—she also felt unusually calm, a new and remarkable sensation for her. She had achieved this through accepting and not reacting to her body's feelings. That process had taken her through becoming conscious of both sensations of pain and emotions of fear that her symptoms had masked and releasing them. Eileen was now aware that her physical symptoms were camouflaging other, deeper layers of experience, and that becoming conscious of these deeper layers was key to her physical improvement.

In our third session, Eileen continued to grow in self-awareness and to develop strategies to help herself heal. While she was lying on the table, I asked her to bring her attention to her right hip, which palpation now told me was more restricted than her left. Eileen was surprised to notice that there was an area the size of a grapefruit in her hip that felt numb. To help her get more in touch with the feeling of that part of her body, I asked her to identify with her right hip and to describe how it felt, using "I" to describe the sensations, as if those sensations had a voice of their own. This was simply a technique to get Eileen more deeply absorbed in her own sensations. By giving Eileen's hip a voice, we were bypassing any temptation on Eileen's part to interpret her sensations rather than feel them directly.

Eileen's right hip told us, "I feel numb." When I asked for how long the hip had been feeling numb, it answered—using Eileen's voice—"For quite a while." Then the hip spontaneously added, "I'm doing a job." Eileen was surprised by this comment and noticed that the idea was new to her, so new that it definitely felt as though it were coming from some part of her that was independent of her conscious mind. Strange as this may sound, it is not at all far-fetched. Scientific evidence indicates that our intelligence is spread throughout the body, not just in the brain alone, and that the feeling processes located in our bodies form part of our subconscious rather than our conscious mind. By activating her own tissue awareness, Eileen was tapping into some of the subconscious processes, thoughts, and emotions that had been removed from her conscious awareness. When subconscious thoughts and emotions become conscious, they feel novel and different to the conscious mind, as if they were coming from someone else.

I asked Eileen to continue staying in touch with her right hip, and I asked her hip, "What kind of job are you doing?" The answer came back immediately: "I'm hiding something." When I asked what the hip was hiding, the answer was "Pain." When I asked what kind of pain, the answer came back: "Emotions." When I asked why the numbness in the right hip was hiding emotions, the answer came back: "Showing emotions is a sign of weakness." Eileen's body was telling her it needed to be numb and in pain as the price it paid for hiding her emotions, and that she needed to hide her emotions because some part of her thought that showing them was a sign of weakness.

An old and powerful part of Eileen—the part that had grown up with Holocaust survivor parents who had lived in dread of the tornado of horror locked inside of them—felt that emotional expression was taboo. In her childhood world, the only way you could be safe was to avoid feelings. The little girl Eileen had rationalized this by deciding that showing emotions was an act of weakness. But as the adult Eileen heard her own body parroting her unconscious childhood convictions, she also had an opportunity to recognize the cost of holding on to those beliefs. That cost was physical pain.

Eileen thought of her own children, whom she encouraged to express themselves freely. She recognized that if she wished them to feel emotionally safe, she would have to model this for them by expressing herself openly around them. That day, Eileen began to shift her worldview and to feel that emotional vulnerability might be a strength worth cultivating rather than a flaw. She admitted that she needed to practice getting in touch with and expressing her feelings. She saw that she needed to learn how to be vulnerable. She realized that there was a link between her physical pain and her fear of emotional self-expression. Finally, she recognized that she could most easily get in touch with her feelings by staying in touch with and feeling her body.

Over time, Eileen worked out a compromise between her anxiety about feeling her emotions and her understanding that defending against feeling them was making her sick. By practicing some of the techniques described in chapter 11, she learned how to use her body awareness to identify how she really felt underneath the brilliant coping exterior that said all was well and that never lost its smile. Eileen worked on expressing how she felt, even though it was scary. She reminded herself that showing emotions could be a sign of strength and self-empowerment. When her chronic pain symptoms flared up, rather than viewing them as a purely physical problem, she asked herself whether she might be having a hard time owning and expressing some feelings. The more Eileen let go into feeling her feelings, the more she could address her real needs and the more her physical symptoms dissipated.

BOB: LETTING GO OF ARMOR

Bob grew up a white Jewish boy in a black big-city ghetto. His father and mother owned a small business in the ghetto, and because the father had a gambling habit, Bob grew up poor. From the time he was a small child, blacks in the neighborhood regularly beat him up. By the age of nine, he had begun training with weights to help him defend himself against the constant danger that surrounded him. He witnessed his parents being held up at gunpoint, was held up several times himself, experienced numerous severe beatings, and learned to fight back hard.

Somehow Bob managed to pull himself out of the ghetto and develop a thriving career. He had learned to keep going at all costs and to survive through anything. The cost of this skill, however, was a complete suppression of his feelings, and by middle age, his body was showing signs of deep wear. Bob came to work with me about a year after he had suddenly and completely collapsed, without warning, in a state of total adrenal exhaustion. Nutrition and lengthy rest had begun to bring him back to life, but he was aware he had a problem. He told me that he lived in an extreme state of tension and was aware of an inability to feel. For example, in his practice as a martial artist, he never felt pain, no matter how violently he was thrown. Bob knew that his early experiences had taught him how to survive pain by suppressing it. But he also recognized intuitively that this skill was endangering his health.

I told Bob that we would work with helping his body relax more and advised him that as that happened, feelings might come up. Bob got onto the bodywork table, and I guided him gently into deeper re-laxation. My hands were drawn like a magnet to his chest. As I held my hands there, I asked him how his body felt. Bob said that his torso, and especially his chest, felt as though it were encased in armor. He had never noticed this before.

Bob stayed present to the armored sensation for a while, absorbing it. Then I asked him if he could feel anything underneath the armor, perhaps a softer area. He said yes, he could feel his softness, but he couldn't show it because of the armor. I asked him if it would be pos-sible to let go of some of the armor—or tension—surrounding his body, and Bob answered adamantly, "Absolutely not!" If he let go of his armor, he might die! It had protected him all his life and was his dearest friend. It may well be that Bob wouldn't have survived as a boy and a young man if he had allowed himself to feel the pain of all the mutilations and beatings he had suffered. But now he was drain-ing his life force through the constant inner demand to be on guard against danger.

Our first session ended with an uneasy truce: the fact that Bob was able for the first time to feel his armor meant that the armor was no longer impenetrable. During our subsequent sessions, Bob's past pain, which had been camouflaged by his armor, came up for release. For example, at one point I felt restrictions in Bob's right shoulder and asked him to become present to that area. Almost immediately, Bob plunged into vivid memories of being beaten in his chest and shoulder and almost killed. As he told me later, he had not felt the pain at the time of the incident, but he had felt it in our session. He yelled and cried through much of the session, at one point screaming out, "I am alive, I am alive, I am alive! I am not dead! You didn't kill me!"

In a series of sessions, Bob relived the physical and emotional pain he had buried inside. As he learned to feel again, he released the ten-sion of protecting himself against his own feelings. He returned to greater health and let go of the driving compulsion that had con-trolled his life.

RECOMMENDATIONS

The more we practice feeling our body, the more in touch we become with our buried emotions. The body walls off buried emotions from consciousness, and the effort of walling them off can be the source of great physical pain. Learning to acknowledge, own, express, and release suppressed emotions can ease chronic pain. The stories in this chapter point to one conclusion: that learning to feel our bodies reduces physical tension and stress by opening up the avenue of suppressed emotional experience. The next chapter explores particular strategies for learning to recognize and own our suppressed emotions.

FURTHER READING

John Upledger, *Your Inner Physician and You* (Berkeley, Calif.: North Atlantic Books, 1991). A very readable introduction to craniosacral therapy by its foremost proponent and founder of the Upledger Institute, one of the world's leading alternative therapy teaching institutes.

11

OWNING BURIED EMOTIONS

Suppose you agree with the idea that chronic pain can result from unacknowledged, unexpressed feelings. Why go through the body to learn to express them? Why can't you just decide to get well by speaking up? In principle, this idea makes sense, but the problem is that unexpressed feelings are largely unconscious; they are feelings we have learned to defend against having. Eileen was not conscious of her deep inner panic, nor of the walls she had put up to avoid her emotions, until she got in touch with her unconscious mind through her body. Bob was not conscious of the tremendous armor he had put on, nor of the deep memories of physical and emotional pain this armor hid, until he too contacted unconscious processes through his body. Similarly, every one of us has disowned feelings—feelings that we have decided to bury rather than to own.

PSYCHOTHERAPY: HELP OR HINDRANCE?

Psychotherapy can certainly be useful. It offers the opportunity to focus directly on your emotional issues and to work with someone who may be gifted in helping you explore yourself. But psychotherapy also has its drawbacks. Most psychotherapists are not professionally trained to recognize the intricate relationships that can link chronic pain, tissue tension, and disowned emotions. In a world in which we overmedicalize chronic pain by treating it as a problem of purely physical origin, this can be a major problem. I myself was in psychotherapy for seven years during the period in which I suffered my most severe bouts of chronic pain. My therapist assumed, as did my doctors, that my pain was a collagen disease pure and simple, unrelated to emotional issues. Partly as a result of this assumption, my therapist was unable to mobilize physical healing for me by helping me gain access to my buried emotions. It took my working with body awareness to begin that process.

Psychotherapy is a form of talk therapy, and its primary approach is to try to stimulate healing through the patient's conscious mind. But while the conscious mind can be an ally, it also blocks subconscious processes that may be key to healing from physical pain. Entrenched in the status quo, the conscious mind is committed to keeping the unconscious out of sight. Therapists face a strong opponent when they engage the mind and its conscious processes in an attempt to evoke unconscious material. The body, in contrast, is the spokesperson for unconscious feelings and experiences. The more we get in touch with it, the more we feel our disowned feelings. Why not use the body as an ally to help a patient gain greater self-awareness?

Most psychotherapists are not trained in the process of helping clients get in touch with their feelings through their bodies. One exception to this rule is the psychotherapist Eugene Gendlin, who developed a technique for integrating body awareness into talk therapy, described in his book *Focusing*. Gendlin engages his clients through talk, but rather than have them *think* about how they feel, he guides them into *feeling* more clearly how they feel by focusing their attention on the *felt sensation* of their bodies. Let's say you are talking to your therapist and you start out by saying "I feel irritable today." Rather than asking you why or how you feel irritable, a therapist trained in Gendlin's technique might ask, "Where or how do you feel that in your body?" Focusing your attention on your body, you might reply, "My chest feels tight," to which the therapist might reply, "Could you stay with that sensation of tightness a bit?" After a while the therapist might ask, "Could you describe how your chest feels now?" You might then say, "The tightness gave way to a feeling of sadness, and I realize I'm sad about an argument I had with a friend of mine yesterday." The therapist might then ask, "Could you stay with that feeling of sadness now?" The session would continue in this manner, taking the client through deeper and deeper layers of feeling.

The fundamental premise of Gendlin's work is that focusing on being present to our body sensations is a more efficient tool for finding our true feelings than thinking about our feelings. Thinking often takes us away from our deeper feelings, whereas the body offers a direct door to the emotions.

Gendlin's approach is extremely useful for contacting buried feelings that may contribute to chronic pain symptoms. Bodywork approaches such as craniosacral therapy add even another dimension: the dimension of touch.

Bodywork of the kind described here is interactive rather than manipulative. The therapist does not do something to the client. Rather, therapist and client cooperate in heightening the client's presence to himself or herself. Bodywork techniques trigger emotional responses and insights by making us more aware of our own tissues and the emotions that reside in those tissues. In the process of contacting and releasing the tissues, you become more present to your subconscious life, more integrated, and more empowered. And since the physical is the mental and the mental is the physical, physical healing work is of necessity emotional healing work and vice versa.

If you suspect that your own chronic pain (or the pain of someone you care for) may be related to unacknowledged feelings, you may wish to seek the help of a qualified craniosacral therapist who works with releasing unconscious emotions. Resources for pursuing this process are found at the end of this chapter.

HOW CAN YOU OWN YOUR EMOTIONS
AND REDUCE YOUR PAIN?

It is not essential to work with a therapist to achieve your own heal-ing. Most of the suggestions that follow offer specific self-help tech-niques for contacting and releasing your emotional core.

1. *Assume that emotional expression is good.* Ask yourself if you are comfortable with emotional self-expression. Many of us are not. We tell ourselves that we are weak, mushy, self-involved, or selfish if we express feelings. We shut down because we fear other people's re-actions. Yet the stronger person is the one who expresses feelings, not the one who can't. When you have a feeling—and especially if you are frightened of expressing it—you need to work on expressing it. If you are with someone, you may need to say, "I'm scared about shar-ing this, and I'm not used to being vulnerable in this way, so please help me. I feel . . ."

Look at any beliefs you have that tell you your emotions are bad, and dare to challenge those beliefs. Good health depends on in-tegrity, as does feeling good about life, and both of these depend on having a rich, expressive emotional life. You figure out who you are and what you want through expressing your emotions. You develop healthy relationships that empower you and the other person, rather than unhealthy relationships that degenerate into subtle or not-so-subtle power struggles, only through expressing emotions. Pain may be your body's way of telling you that you are not being true to your-self because you are sacrificing too much of yourself to a belief system you learned or to the needs of others.

2. *Use breath awareness to enhance your emotional awareness.* Chapters 4 and 5 describe the use of breath awareness as a vital tool for reducing pain. Breath awareness—including meditation on the breath and daily awareness of how you are breathing—also plays an essential role in helping you become more aware of your emotions. When you meditate or breathe deeply, easily, and regularly, you release tensions in your body, and this gives your emotions the opportunity to rise to the

surface. Deeper emotions need space to become conscious. Breath awareness calms your system down enough that you begin to become more aware of your inner life and less involved in the stresses and strains of the endless running around that takes you out of yourself.

I have taught breath awareness for many years, and almost invariably students in my classes find it extremely pleasurable and relaxing. Yet many people have difficulty using breath awareness in their daily lives. If we are not used to breathing our way through life, it is difficult to change. Learning to be at ease with our breath also makes us more self-aware, and this challenges us to be at ease with ourselves and the way we feel. If you need to avoid your feelings, or if you are scared of your feelings, you will impede your breathing in order to keep them buried. But if you understand that breath awareness is your pathway to self-awareness, self-acceptance, and freedom from pain, you will ride through the emotions that come up as you breathe and will learn to honor what they tell you. Learning to feel and enjoying the process of feeling—even difficult feelings—is the essence of living fully. When we feel deeply, we are alive. When we don't feel deeply, we fill our lives with substitutes that don't really satisfy us. One of the consequences can be chronic pain.

Breathe, feel your feelings as you do this, and have the courage to own how you feel. Later chapters will guide you through how to use your feelings more effectively to negotiate your way through life. This process has to begin, however, with owning rather than disowning your feelings.

3. *Slow down to be present.* When we are present to ourselves, we can feel our emotions. The most important single technique for being present is to slow down. Breath awareness helps you with this. Learning to value being present to yourself more than getting things done also helps. Ours is a society in motion, and constant motion is a universally accepted form of compulsive behavior. It is difficult to slow down, even though you may complain about the fast pace of life. Staying in motion keeps us from feeling, and that in turn helps us to avoid responsibility for our lives. Eileen stayed in constant motion and was a "good" provider, wife, and mother. But she was out of

touch with herself, was driven by fear, and sacrificed herself and her health to the demands of what she thought she was supposed to do. My colleague kept on coping with a heavy schedule, and though this seemed necessary, it also effectively kept him from knowing his deeper feelings and moving fully through his experiences. Lucia denied her right to feel her feelings by continually focusing on what she had to get done for her husband. And Bob kept his plate overfull to avoid deep feelings of pain. We live in a society that emphasizes doing, performing, and speed, but the price we pay is chronic tension, pain, and emotional impoverishment.

The clearest indicator of being overfocused on what we have to accomplish and lacking presence to ourselves, is an overactive mind. Our mind chatters at us constantly, giving us lots of things to think about and reasons not to feel. For example, when we wake up in the morning, the first thing we do is recite to ourselves the long list of things we have to accomplish during the day. Or we return from an evening out and spend an hour obsessing over what kind of impression we made on our colleagues. Or we realize in the midst of a conversation that we haven't registered a word of what someone was saying to us because we were so absorbed in our own internal monologue.

Be aware that when your mind talks to you constantly and you are continually focused on what you have to get done next, you are in a state of stress, and that stress creates pain. Remember that the quality of your breathing, your level of muscle tension, your mental state, and your emotional state, all correlate (see chapter 4, page 53). When your mind is full of chatter, your breathing is shallow, your body is tense, and you are driven by negative emotions such as fear and anxiety. When your mind becomes overactive, what you actually need to do in order to focus better is to *slow down*. You do this simply by becoming present to your body's sensations, by focusing your attention *inwardly* and nonjudgmentally on how you feel, rather than *outwardly* on what you have to do.

If you stop and pay attention to your body sensations when you find your mind racing, you will probably notice that your body is tense: your shoulders are tight, your breathing is constricted, your gut is clenched, and so on. Your body's tension is an accurate indicator that you are out of touch with yourself and that you are being driven by emotions of fear. Tune in to your body, and make your first priority releasing body tension. Releasing body tension will always guide you in a better direction, because it directs you to let go of the anxiety or anger that may be driving you. In doing so, it also eases physical pain and calms you so that you can focus more effectively on defining your true priorities.

4. *Once a day, feel your feelings in your body.* Each day, set aside a specific time to feel your feelings in your body. This practice will develop your ability to stay more in touch with your feeling life. When you go to bed at night—and also at various points during the day—relax and slow down your left brain for a few minutes by following your breathing. Then take five to ten minutes to feel your feelings. To do this, begin by scanning your body.

Let your attention be drawn to an area that is calling out to you. Be present to that part of yourself. Let it feel however it feels. Breathe into it. Absorb how that part of your body feels. Do not expect to feel anything in particular. Just honor however that part of your body feels. Be interested in it. Stay with this process for a few minutes, and you will notice the sensation gradually evolving. You may simply feel changing physical sensations. You may also feel emotions that you were not previously aware of. Allow this process to unfold, without prejudgment as to which direction it will take. Observe and appreciate any emotions that emerge, and do not try to avoid or change any emotions or sensations. If you feel pain, allow it to pass through. If you feel anger or grief or fear, breathe and allow yourself to observe and experience the feeling.

At first, you will find it difficult to stay with your felt sensations. Your mind will wander. Whenever you become aware of your mind wandering, just return to being present to how your body feels. You will become increasingly in touch with your body's sensations and your emotions.

5. *Let your body's feelings talk to you.* You can enhance the

power of the practice described above by reporting your sensations and emotions out loud as you experience them. I encouraged Eileen to do this by asking her to give parts of her body a voice and then to describe how a part felt by having that body part say, "I feel . . ." In the same way, in your daily practice of feeling your feelings in your body, you may, for example, be drawn to a tension in your knee. You can then explore this feeling further, saying, for example, "I feel tight . . . I feel tense . . . I feel all bottled up . . . " Continue this process, allowing yourself to explore and to describe what you feel for five minutes or more. By verbalizing how your body feels, you enable yourself to move more quickly from physical felt sensations to emotional sensations and to delve more deeply into yourself. Verbalization also helps you stay focused and prevents your mind from wandering. You may gain invaluable insights through this process.

6. *Write your feelings in a journal.* In order to express your feelings to others, you must learn first to express them to yourself. The more you articulate your feelings to yourself, the clearer they will be to you and the more you will trust them. Verbalizing your feelings out loud—as in No. 5—will help you, but it will also help you to keep a journal. Write in this journal daily. Start each entry with "I feel." Write a page or more, staying with the felt sensation of your body as you write rather than trying to think about and analyze how you feel. Don't worry about whether what you are writing is good or makes sense. It is for your eyes and your eyes alone. Just write. Discover yourself.

If you have not worked with journal writing before, you may wish to consult Julia Cameron's excellent book *The Artist's Way* to help mobilize your writing process.

7. *Consider seeking the help of a bodywork professional.* If you have long-term chronic pain, feel that you may be out of touch with your deeper emotions, and think that you need the help of a professional, consider seeking the assistance of someone skilled in the emotional release work that is an integral aspect of craniosacral therapy. You may want to ask bodyworkers in your area whether they know any skilled craniosacral therapists. In order to practice craniosacral ther-

apy, a therapist must be a licensed bodyworker: for example, a physical therapist, occupational therapist, massage therapist, chiropractor, or movement therapist. You may also call the Upledger Institute in Florida, which is a leading center for training in craniosacral therapy. The institute will provide you with reliable referrals to practitioners in your area. Contact information is provided at the end of this chapter.

RECOMMENDATIONS

Learn to own your emotions. First, assume that emotional expression is good. Second, use breath awareness to enhance your emotional awareness. Third, slow down to become more present. Fourth, practice feeling the feelings in your body. Fifth, let your body's feelings talk to you. Sixth, write your feelings. Seventh, seek the help of a bodywork professional. The recommended reading and practitioner contacts below will aid in your further exploration of these areas.

Some emotions are buried deeper than others and can cause deeper, more intractable pain. The next chapter addresses this conflict and its resolution.

FURTHER READING

Julia Cameron, *The Artist's Way* (New York: G. P. Putnam, 1992). An excellent guide to writing your way to freer self-expression.

Eugene Gendlin, *Focusing* (New York: Bantam, 1979). A guide to exploring your emotions by focusing on the felt sensations of the body.

PRACTITIONERS

To find out about craniosacral therapy practitioners in your area, contact the Upledger Institute at (800) 233-5880 or through the institute's Web site, www.upledger.com.

12

EMOTIONAL CONFLICT, PAIN, AND SELF-EMPOWERMENT

Our feelings are our life force. When we discount, dismiss, or suppress our feelings, the consequence can be chronic pain. When this happens, the chances are that deep forces are at play that are keeping us out of touch with ourselves. As the stories of Lucia, my colleague, Eileen, and Bob imply, we can feel uncomfortable about our emotions. The more uncomfortable we feel, the harder our feelings are to admit and the more potential damage they can wreak on our bodies. This chapter explores more fully how conflict over our emotions creates chronic pain, as well as some of the reasons why that conflict may develop. The subsequent chapter looks at tools for resolving conflict and promoting freedom from pain.

CONFLICT, ANGER, AND VIOLATED BOUNDARIES

When I was ill and disabled by chronic pain, my self-healing began as I learned how to identify sensations of neuromuscular tension in my body and release them. The more clearly I felt my body, however, the more my emotions began to come to the surface and the more I noticed a connection between acknowledging uncomfortable emotions and a reduction of pain.

The first series of experiences that made this connection between emotional conflict and pain crystal clear to me began a week after my father died. An evening Mass was scheduled for my father at St. Patrick's Cathedral in New York City. I was to join my sisters and step-mother there at five in the afternoon. When I woke up in the morning, I was feeling quite well. It was early in March, and I was preparing my garden for spring planting. As I lifted a forty-pound bag of compost out of the trunk of my car, I felt a minor twinge in my back. I dismissed it as insignificant and went on with my work. By the time I left for the funeral Mass, my back was stiff. The next morning, I was too sore to get out of bed. I decided that I had sprained my back in lifting the compost bag the day before. The pain would no doubt dissipate within a few days. But it didn't. A week later, I was just as sore.

Meanwhile, I mourned my father's passing despite a history with him that was not particularly happy. My parents had divorced when I was nine, and my father had remarried and fathered another family, which had become his primary concern. This had caused me to feel abandoned by him. My father was also insecure, inarticulate with his feelings, unable to give and receive freely, and quick to criticize. My child's heart needed and adored him, however, and hoped he held me in a special place in his heart. I did everything I could to please him and gain his love. Now that he was gone, I grieved for him—and grieved. Meanwhile, my back ached—and ached.

A few days later, an old friend of the family came around and we started talking. Unexpectedly, I found myself expressing anger toward my father. I had never done this before! But now the words of anger seemed to fly out of my mouth. Even though I knew that my father had been incapable of emotional warmth and had long ago excused him for his weaknesses, now I was nonetheless angry that he had rarely if ever reached out to me. I was angry that he had left everything in his last will and testament to his second family and nothing to the three children of his first family. I was angry that he had failed throughout our relationship to remember my birthday. I was angry that he had neglected to attend my college graduation at Harvard or to be at my wedding. My disappointment and rage poured out as my friend and I sat across from each other over dinner. At the end of dinner, I paid for the meal and rose to get my coat. With surprise, I noticed that my back felt much better. Over the next few days, my back continued to improve, and a week later my symptoms were gone.

What had happened? The answer lay in my history. I had learned never to express feelings of anger toward my father. Our relationship had been so precarious that I had intuitively realized that the only way I could maintain any connection with him was to behave in a way that would please him. All my life he had failed me in so many of the small daily rituals that make up a secure loving connection. I had never been able to rely on a warm hug and kiss for a greeting, let alone on a dad who would join me in my triumphs and my trials or cheer me on. From the time I was nine, when my parents divorced, I felt I had to take care of his emotional needs rather than my own because he was so fragile. I had to do everything to keep him from abandoning me more than he already had. And so I had repressed my anger, a natural response to my feelings of rejection and mistreatment. My feelings were too dangerous to own.

My childhood had taught me that other people's feelings were more important than my own. When my father died, however, my insides—my feeling life—finally felt safer. Here was an opportunity to explode with all my withheld rage, and without fear of retaliation or rejection.

My subconscious mind saw my father's death as an opportunity to own all the feelings I had been afraid of expressing. My father could no longer abandon me because he was already gone. Yet my conscious mind was used to denying the reality of my anger. I had to be a good girl! My tissues were used to holding on tight in the effort of suppressing the rage that was taboo. The result of the conflict between my exploding anger and my need to be good was an intolerable tension in my body. That conflict caused my back to go into spasm. When I finally let the anger through, owned it, and gave myself permission to feel emotions that I had viewed as so dangerous that I couldn't even recognize them as mine, the conflict eased, and so did my back pain.

Since that experience, I have many times noticed that I begin to suffer from back pain when I am having difficulty expressing my feelings and claiming appropriate boundaries. This has generally happened in situations where I have given too much authority to someone else, whether that person was my employer, a colleague, a family member, or my partner. I had become so used to denying my own needs that it took numerous experiences to recognize when I had overextended myself for someone else. Back pain was my signal that I was out of balance. Getting past the pain required me to own my own anger, an anger that was a natural result of giving too little priority to taking care of myself. The more I learned to own my anger and state my boundaries, the less frequently my back bothered me.

My own history and attitudes are far from unique. I learned from childhood that anger was not a nice emotion and that if it were expressed the punishment for its expression would be severe. Many people feel that it is not nice to be angry or that it places a black mark on their character. In addition, when anger begins to emerge, it is tempting to tell ourselves that we shouldn't be angry or that maybe things are different from the way we see them. Perhaps we are wrong! Or maybe we will soon feel differently from the way we feel right now! Such equivocations express one thing only: fear. Fear of owning our own experience. If we engage in these equivocations, chronic pain remains. That pain expresses the intense stress we are under, living in fear and bottling up the anger that is seeking to come to our defense.

Anger can be dysfunctional, but it can also be healthy. Healthy anger is an organic acknowledgment of boundary violation, of the fact that we are in a situation that does not work for us. Anger comes up because we have stayed in that situation too long and things need to change. When we can own our anger, we can leave the situation or change it—or, if appropriate, change ourselves.

Anger becomes explosive only when we can't own it. Then it builds up inside until the pressure becomes unbearable. At this point, we either act it out against other people, usually inappropriately, or turn it against ourselves. If we act it out against other people, we blame them for our emotional state rather than taking responsibility for our lives and initiating necessary changes. When we blame or hold others responsible, we initiate a mutually self-destructive cycle of emotional abuse. When we turn anger against ourselves rather than acting it out on others, we foster a different kind of self-destructive cycle: a cycle of increasing discomfort, pain, and disease.

Your challenge is to own the strength of how you feel—not simply exploding but giving yourself permission to feel how you feel no matter how those feelings affect those around you or how others perceive you. Repressed anger reflects the fact that you have disempowered yourself. In order to own your own feelings, release your tension, and work with your feelings constructively, you have to be willing to own the way you feel, *even though others may disagree*.

You have to be able to say "No," to differ. In my own case, for example, I had to be able both to acknowledge my anger and pain over my father's treatment and, when I could do it without recriminations, share honestly with my stepmother and siblings how painful my father's behavior had been for me, rather than defending him and making it all right.

JESSICA: DISEMPOWERMENT AND PAIN

I have worked with many clients whose pain was an expression of their own lack of personal power and whose journey out of pain involved a struggle to feel and accept the legitimacy of their anger and then to change their situation. Jessica, whose background had some similarities to my own, came to see me, complaining of sciatic pain. Jessica was engaged to be married but was quite anxious about this. Forty years old, she had never been married, and even though she loved her fiancé, Don, she associated marriage with being confined and with having to give up part of herself. Her fiancé seemed emotionally unexpressive, which reminded her of her father. Jessica made most of the effort in the relationship with her fiancé. She drove from New York to Boston every weekend to visit him. She had put up her house for sale, was willing to rebuild her business in his hometown, and was trying to act the future stepmother with Don's son. Jessica felt somewhat resentful at Don's lack of appreciation, but she didn't dare share this with him.

Jessica was overextending and draining herself. She was not getting back as much as she was giving. As soon as I suggested to Jessica that she was draining herself, she recalled a visit to a psychic years before. The psychic had told her that her father had drained her because she had always felt she had to protect him. Jessica's father had not been there for her when she was young and had refused to contribute to her college tuition. These material failures had also been a form of emotional abandonment. But Jessica had not reacted by distancing herself from her father. He was all she had, and she wanted his love. So she bottled up her feelings, stretched herself for her father, and was grateful for anything she got.

Jessica remembered the one time in her life when she had asked her father for money—a loan of three thousand dollars—and he had actually given it to her. She began to cry tears of gratitude for the love he showed her in this act. Anyone else could have seen, however, that Jessica's gratitude was exaggerated and inappropriate, given her long history of paternal neglect. She cried because she was grateful for crumbs. This tendency kept her in situations that exhausted her. She had to give so much to get a minuscule return.

Jessica and I looked for parallels between her relationship with her father and her relationship with Don. Jessica decided to risk asking for more from Don. She feared that if she asked for more or established stronger boundaries, things would fall apart. It was her fear—hidden behind her great coping skills and combined with resentment over the effort that she had to make to get a response from Don—that was feeding her back pain. She felt disempowered.

It was scary for Jessica to assert her own needs more forcefully with Don. She had to confront her fear that she would lose him if she spoke up for herself. But doing so was also exhilarating because she felt more in control of her life. Eventually, Jessica decided that Don could not give her what she needed, and it was she, rather than he, who put an end to the relationship. By that time, her back pain was gone.

TRADITIONAL MEDICINE, EMOTIONAL CONFLICT, AND CHRONIC PAIN

Few medical specialists consider how large a role emotional conflict can play in the etiology of chronic pain. Within the medical profession, John Sarno, author of *Mind over Back Pain* and *Healing Back Pain*, stands as the exception to this rule. Professor of Clinical rehabilitation medicine at the New York University School of Medicine and a physician at the University's Medical Center, Sarno has treated thousands of back patients for more than twenty years. Although he began his work within the traditional, physiological approach to back pain, he was troubled by the fact that treatments that addressed purely structural problems were not particularly successful with patients. Sarno's research led him to the conclusion that structural problems were rarely the key issue. Rather, he decided that the primary cause of chronic pain was what he called tension myositis syndrome, or chronic tension in the musculature related to reduced blood flow to the muscles. According to Sarno, this muscle tension and oxygen debt cause pain.

Sarno describes tension myositis syndrome as a stress response that reflects suppressed anxiety or anger. His treatment method is primarily educational. Patients learn about the relationship between pain, tension, and suppressed feelings. This relieves them from fear about their physical condition and from overfocusing on pursuing a purely medical approach to their pain. Instead, they focus on addressing the issues in their lives that are causing stress. Improvement is often rapid, and Sarno has helped thousands of people reduce their chronic pain.

Sarno's method is particularly useful for patients who fulfill three conditions. First, the underlying cause of their pain syndrome lies in conflicts and suppressed feelings. Second, they not only have not received benefit from traditional medicine but also in some cases have actually worsened, because traditional medical diagnoses have stimulated their anxiety and sense of disempowerment over what seems to be a physical problem over which they have no control. Third, once their attention is drawn to the possibility that emotional conflict is the cause of their pain, they are able to *recognize, acknowledge,* and *deal with* the conflict effectively.

Jessica was one person who was able quickly to recognize and address her conflicts and resolve her pain through effective action. Many people can do this, but many cannot. They cannot consciously recognize what is bothering them emotionally simply as a result of being told that they are in conflict, because their emotions are too well defended. Such people need instead to begin by discovering the feelings that are so deeply suppressed in the unconscious that they are not available to the type of approach used by Sarno. They can do this, as in the cases of Lucia, Eileen, and Bob, through training in body awareness, which helps trigger recognition of the conflicts that lie below the surface of consciousness. Sometimes, as the following case of Marilyn shows, further professional intervention through intensive craniosacral therapy also opens the door to dealing with hidden conflicts.

MARILYN: WHEN DISEMPOWERMENT IS CALLED LOVE

Marilyn was referred to me because of chronic neck pain, as well as pain in one of her hips. We began our work together with meditative breathing, body scans, and alignment training, all of which helped her feel better physically. During the process of this work, Marilyn also reported that while focusing on diaphragmatic breathing, she had spontaneously had memories of being physically abused as a child. Difficult memories—along with the emotions associated with them—were emerging through the deep relaxation work as the tensions that held them back dissolved. I suspected that there were further emotional issues involved in Marilyn's pain.

Marilyn gradually became more in tune with her body. One day while she was on the bodywork table, she reported feeling as though she had a terrible weight on her chest. I had placed my hands in that area. I asked her to see if she could stay present to the feeling in her chest. Marilyn did this, and in less than a minute, she was sobbing and sobbing. She recognized that her tears were about her sister, who had died of ovarian cancer. Her sister had had difficulty accepting any expression of emotion, and Marilyn had been unable to express her feelings for her or to cry in front of her. This had been very painful, and she felt she had been unable to establish an emotional connection with her sister as she was dying.

As Marilyn sobbed, she revealed that the same thing had also happened when her mother had died. Like her sister, Marilyn's mother had had a long-standing history of rejecting any expression of feeling on Marilyn's part. As a child, Marilyn had had to go into the bathroom to cry because her mother objected to her tears. On the table, Marilyn's pain eased as she let out the grief of a lifetime.

Before Marilyn left that day, I encouraged her to recognize that her feelings were not wrong. She had not been at fault in feeling her grief. Marilyn had disempowered herself as a child by feeling she was at fault because others could not accept her emotions. This feeling had reinforced her emotional suppression and reduced her self-esteem, all of which had contributed to the stress that fed her pain. When Marilyn left that day, she felt more comfortable about having permission to feel her feelings. Her hip and neck also felt somewhat better.

The next time Marilyn came for a session, she told me she felt like crying and that she thought her grief was related to her mother's death. I invited her to lie down on the bodywork table, so that we could process her feelings more deeply. When I palpated her body, I was immediately drawn to the area around Marilyn's liver. I was surprised at this, since in acupuncture theory, the liver is traditionally associated with anger. I said nothing, however, and let Marilyn begin her process. Marilyn began to cry, saying she felt terrible because she couldn't feel her love for her mother. This bothered her deeply. I asked her to tell me more about her feelings toward her mother, and she said that as a child she had been "dishonest" to her mother. When I asked her what she meant, she said that her mother had not liked feelings and had gotten angry readily, so she had had to watch out for what she said. Marilyn said she had tailored her behavior to fit what her mother would accept, so that she could feel connected to her. Then Marilyn also said she felt that she had "betrayed" her mother toward the end of her life by putting her in a hospice. Her mother had been very angry about this, but Marilyn had felt she had no choice, since she could not handle the care of her mother on her own.

I commented to Marilyn that she had unjustly accused herself twice, once of being "dishonest" and once of "betraying" her mother. I suggested that the fault was perhaps not her own and that in accusing herself she was taking responsibility for her mother's demands. I asked Marilyn if she could now be "honest" and imagine saying to her mother all the things she had never been able to say to her. Marilyn's first words were gentle. She told her mother she missed and loved her. But soon her tone changed, and anger poured out: anger that her mother had neglected her, anger that her mother had not come to her wedding, anger that her mother had favored Marilyn's stepfather, who had been abusive to Marilyn.

Marilyn had spent a lifetime learning to see herself as the problem. She had labeled herself as unloving because she couldn't match up to her mother's demands. She had also spent years trying hard to relate to and express love to family members who wouldn't relate to her. Inevitably, underneath her feelings of love there were feelings of abandonment, rejection, and anger.

In our previous work together, Marilyn had already connected to her body enough to be able to acknowledge some of her deeper feelings. Yet she was also used to defending against her deeper feelings, especially when they involved resentment and anger. And so the first thing that she did when she lay down was to go into a defensive posture that was familiar to her: feeling the need to love her mother more deeply, to be more connected, and to accuse herself if she could not feel this connection.

Three things helped Marilyn break through her defenses. First, she had already absorbed the idea from the previous session that the conflict with her sister and mother had not necessarily been her fault. Her mother and sister had contributed to making it hard for her to express her emotions. Second, when I questioned her perception of herself as "dishonest," and as "betraying" her mother, I helped her to re-frame her experience and accept emotions of anger that she was afraid to acknowledge. Third, I had palpated her liver—a traditional seat for feelings of anger—as the primary restriction that day, and laid my hands over that area. My touch triggered Marilyn's awareness of subliminal feelings of anger and encouraged her to express them.

In the weeks that followed, Marilyn discovered buried wells of anger that, when she allowed them to burst out, relieved her both emotionally and physically. Each time a session started, she felt un-comfortable but not consciously aware of any outstanding issue. Each time, as she lay on the table and we worked with palpation and dia-logue, she would get in touch with deep feelings of pain about mis-treatment and abuse she had suffered as a child. Each time, she felt relief only after she *fully and vociferously acted out her anger:* by yelling, thumping, screaming, and in one way or another saying, "I am not going to let you get me down! No! No! No!" Over time, her neck and hip bothered her less and less.

THE POWER OF VENTING

Marilyn's story exemplifies what Peter Levine, in *Waking the Tiger,* talks about when he says that life trauma can cause us to freeze. When this happens, we can unfreeze from our paralysis only by mo-bilizing an extremely strong response that wakes us from our paralysis. Freezing is an intense stress reaction based in nature. Animals often freeze when in extreme danger, for example, when pinned by a lion. Humans freeze too. When we freeze, we are completely disempow-ered. To release yourself from an emotional trauma and to return to a sense of control over your destiny, of personal empowerment, you have to have a powerful *action* response. You have to learn how to move into action again. This learning must be forceful. Marilyn needed to explore and explode into her anger again and again and to express it as powerfully as she could, sometimes thrashing and kicking and often yelling, to persuade herself of her own right to be free of the shackles of her family. She had to vent her feelings in no uncertain terms. She had to voice her anger repeatedly in order to get past the prohibition that told her that anytime she felt anger, she was a bad person. Most of all, she had to vent her anger as part of learning and owning that she could differ from others. She could hold to her own feelings and opinions, regardless of whether others agreed with or accepted her views.

To empower herself, Marilyn had to learn to say "No!" Once Marilyn allowed herself to own her feelings sufficiently to feel safe with them, once she had vented fully, she could begin to address her conflicts with her family without feeling disempowered or controlled. Her back pain then went away completely.

Like Marilyn, I learned from personal experience that when we have repressed our feelings, we may have to practice feeling their validity and reality by expressing them powerfully over and over. Strongly and repeatedly venting my anger in private enabled me to empower myself and to recognize and assert my boundaries. In healing from my wounds over my father, I spent days where I would take my tennis racket and beat on my sofa, yelling at my father and demanding to know how he could possibly have treated his daughter the way he had treated me! This relieved a large backlog of pent-up pain and helped me recognize the importance of my feelings. When I felt back pain in a work situation where I was being insufficiently assertive, I would walk up and down a quiet street, venting my frustration and insisting to myself that I wouldn't take it anymore. Only once I had fully vented my feelings could I feel sufficiently empowered and in my own truth to begin to strategize how to change the situation that was oppressing me, without blowing up at or blaming others but with clarity and self-assertion.

Marilyn's story and my own demonstrate the types of situations in which Dr. Sarno's purely psychological approach to back pain, valuable as it is, may not work. When a person has strong conflicts over establishing boundaries, it may not be enough to suggest that repressed feelings—in particular, repressed anger—are the reason for his or her chronic pain. Those feelings may be too deeply buried. In such cases, bodywork such as craniosacral therapy, which engages the emotional subconscious through the tissues, can prove invaluable. A person may also need to vent emotions repeatedly, so that he or she can get a clearer sense of the legitimacy of his or her own feelings and of his or her ability to take control over his or her own life.

There is another lesson in Marilyn's story, as in my own, a lesson that holds almost universally for chronic pain when that pain results from unconscious conflict. In order to deal successfully with conflict and to move toward greater health, we have to release ourselves from the strangleholds of *obligation* and *guilt.*

HOW A SENSE OF OBLIGATION AND GUILT DISEMPOWERS YOU

Marilyn is typical of many chronic pain victims: she was holding herself down through feelings of obligation and guilt—obligation to give her mother and sister what they wanted and guilt over her own feelings when her spirit rebelled in anger. Feelings of obligation and guilt tend to arise wherever our well-being is overly dependent on responding to others' needs. Since as children we are all dependent on our parents, many of us develop strong feelings of obligation and guilt. Direct or indirect parental prohibitions tell us what we should and shouldn't do, when we are good and when we are bad. Education and religious training add to the weight of our obligation and guilt by giving us standards of right and wrong and requiring us to live by them.

The problem with feelings of obligation and guilt is that their legitimacy comes from the outside: they represent a code that is externally imposed rather than chosen out of some internal, organic sense of rightness. This places our sense of obligation in direct conflict with our ability to listen to our own inner voice.

One of my clients, a highly successful businessman, suffers from periodic mild low back pain and bone spurs of the cervical vertebrae. Well educated, Joseph is by nature gentle, considerate, and generous. He is also Roman Catholic, raised by Catholic parents and educated in Catholic schools. A strong moral code based on obligation and duty has been drummed into him from infancy. As a result, Joseph sometimes has difficulty establishing proper boundaries. When he does, his back reacts.

At one point, Joseph decided to give a large gift to his daughter, to help her build her business. In the process of negotiations with his daughter, however, her husband stepped into the picture and, with an aggressive stance, decided to take over the negotiations and demand more for his wife, on terms that would also allow him to create a business for himself. Joseph's Catholic background had taught him to be of service and always to look for faults in himself rather than in the other person when conflict developed. Joseph therefore failed to object to his son-in-law's takeover of the talks and failed to question the tone of his approach. He couldn't help but become angry, however, and his back began to ache. It was only when, in conversation over the situation, he realized that his son-in-law's behavior was an inappropriate response to a generous gift, that he was able to speak up and tell the man in no uncertain terms that he was overstepping his limits. When he did this, his back pain and neck tension dissipated. He had listened to his own inner sense of what was right for him rather than to the externally imposed voice of a self-denying superego.

Feelings of obligation and guilt typically have a "should" attached to them. For example, you would like to read a book, but you "should" go visit a friend or relative in need. You would like a family member to clean up the dishes after you made dinner, but you "should" be willing to do it yourself. You would like to spend some time by yourself, but you "should" attend an event with your spouse. The "should" list goes on and on, and so does your sense of obligation.

Focusing on your sense of obligation can keep you out of touch with your own needs, as in the cases of Marilyn and Jessica, and lead you into a life of outright fear. I once worked with a woman whose life was dominated by her obsession over what she "should" do. Should she go out to lunch with a friend who had called, even though she didn't want to? Should she be on a college board that had expressed interest in her participation? Should she return the call of a friend, even though right now she had nothing to say? Should she buy a green or a lavender dress for the party she was attending? What would people think? This woman never asked herself what she *wanted* to do, only what she *should* do. The consequence was, first, that she felt ambivalent, and therefore resentful, about whatever she did, because she was never sure that she wanted to do what she did. Her ambivalence fed her tension. Second, she was driven by fear. When we guide ourselves by an external standard of right and wrong, rather than developing our own internal standard, we live in fear. After all, we could be wrong! The consequence for this client was extreme stress, which manifested itself in such deep tension that her body had become seriously rigid and inflexible.

When our dominant guide becomes a sense of obligation, we do things because we feel we have to, not because we want to. We don't enjoy our lives, and we feel out of control. We are disempowered, even though it is no one but ourselves who is making the decisions about what we are going to do.

Healthy feelings of obligation grow out of desire. They express a sense of deep commitment that forms part of the pleasure we get out of life. For example, a mother's feelings of obligation for her child are generally of this kind. She often sacrifices her immediate personal needs and interests for the sake of the child. She does this because her love for the child and the child's growth give her a deeper satisfaction. We all need this form of obligation in our lives.

Unhealthy feelings of obligation, however, do not yield genuine satisfaction. We may obtain the superficial pleasure of feeling that we are a good person because we are doing what we think we are supposed to do. But we give responsibility for our decisions to society, convention, morality, the boss, or family members. We avoid taking responsibility for ourselves. But it is only by taking personal responsibility for our choices that we feel empowered.

An unhealthy sense of obligation can make you sick. You hand over your decisions to an external arbiter, but then you resent the loss of control it entails. You disempower yourself, even as you rage against your own disempowerment. This inevitably puts you into deep conflict, a conflict that can express itself as pain.

Jane came to visit me complaining of chronic migraines that had begun five years before, after she and her only son had become estranged. Her son had initiated the separation, and they had not spoken since that time. Jane soon admitted to feeling extremely angry at her son. After all, she had spent eighteen years doting on him, and to be rewarded with coldness and hostility was too painful for words. But Jane also felt terribly guilty about her anger and hated herself for it. In Jane's mind, it simply was not acceptable to feel the way she did. As she put it, "I'm Irish, and Irish people have to be loyal to the family." In Jane's world, displays of anger against a family member simply were not okay. No matter what someone in the family did, the tribe had to stick together. Even if family members weren't sticking together in reality, they at least had to appear to do so. In Jane's case, that meant no overt displays of feeling against her son. I have seen other persons who are strongly identified with their clan even refuse to deal with incest and physical abuse in their families for similar reasons: addressing these issues openly would mean violating the obligation to be loyal to the clan.

Jane had felt such intense pain over her son's behavior that she had thought of removing him from her will, but when she had broached the subject to her relatives, they had reacted in horror. "You can't do that!" And so Jane was doing what she felt she ought to do. Meanwhile, she secretly seethed on the inside and then hated herself. It was no wonder she had chronic migraines.

Jane was not able to look at how she might heal from the pain of her son's abandonment: most likely by openly airing her feelings and making decisions on that basis. Unfortunately, she defined herself in terms of how her family thought she should behave. She was so embedded in looking at what her family thought was right and wrong that she could not admit to or express her deeper feelings. You can't resolve what you can't admit to. You just go round and round. This stalemate was the cause of Jane's physical pain. The last I heard of her, she was still in debilitating pain and still taking heavy doses of medication to manage that pain.

A few years ago, a woman named Pam came to a lecture series on chronic pain that I was offering at Stamford Hospital in Stamford, Connecticut. After hearing some of my comments on the relationship between chronic stress and pain, she scheduled a visit with me. She had been receiving physical therapy for months without substantial benefit and was sure her fibromyalgia was stress-related. We worked together briefly, and the next week she called to tell me her headaches had disappeared for the first time in months. She did not come back, however, until another year had passed.

When Pam returned, she told me she had almost died in the interim because she had not been able consistently to let go of her own stress patterns. She had been hospitalized several times for pain, severe bronchial infections, adrenal exhaustion, and thyroid problems. As we spoke, she told me she had reached the point of realizing that her sense of guilt and obligation was killing her. Raised by an extremely narcissistic mother, she had learned to serve Mommy's needs first. In the past few years, she had visited her mother in her nursing home two to three times a week, no matter how heavy her own schedule was and despite the travel time involved and the fact that her mother never expressed appreciation for her. Mother came first! In addition, she was married to an aggressive, go-getter husband, had at his request joined his business as its primary sales representative many years before, and had for several decades worked sixty hours a week at a job she hated. She had been filled with a rage that she couldn't express, a rage that is an automatic expression of self-suppression in the name of doing one's duty. Pam had modeled herself along the lines of what her husband asked of her, without considering her right or need to define her own life. Finally, at the age of fifty-six, with multiple physical problems, her life itself was in danger. Pam began to improve only when she faced the fact that she had to give up her guilt or die. She reduced her visits to her mother, told her husband she had to quit her job with his company, convinced him to sell the business, and began a new life. Slowly, her pain receded.

If you are suffering from chronic pain, you may have to look at your feelings of obligation and guilt and see where you are violating your inner needs in the name of a social norm. Strategies for doing this are included in the next chapter.

RECOMMENDATIONS

The process of healing from chronic pain is a process of personal empowerment. The key element is learning that you have the right to say "No!" The right to say "No" is simply the right to own our differences from others and to establish our own boundaries, even and especially if those boundaries do not meet the requirements of those around us. The right to say "No" is the right to disagree, to feel the way you uniquely feel, and to claim the truth that is uniquely yours. To reclaim your right to your feelings, their rightness for you, does not mean that your feelings are right and another person's feelings are wrong. But it does mean that your feelings are yours and that you must begin by respecting them in order to guide your life in the direction that is appropriate for you. By owning your feelings, saying that they are correct for you just because they are yours, you empower yourself, stand up for yourself, and find a more secure footing. It's no wonder that chronic pain of the muscles, joints, and bones dissolves. You can now stand on your own two feet. You can be who you are.

Health is vitally dependent on owning who you are, even at the price of differing. Physical health is closely aligned with individuation, the process of maturation through which you learn to take full responsibility for the choices you make. Individuation requires the ability to say "No," since "No" is also the foundation of a healthy "Yes." But while this is easily said, how is it done in practice? Strategies for owning your power, for learning to say "No," form the subject of the next chapter.

FURTHER READING

Caroline Myss, *Anatomy of the Spirit* (New York: Harmony Books, 1996). A groundbreaking book by a renowned medical intuitive on the intimate links between illness and feelings of personal disempowerment.

John Sarno, *Mind over Back Pain* (New York: Berkley, 1982). In this concise, simply written book, Dr. John Sarno presents and elegantly substantiates his theory that tension is the primary cause of chronic pain.

13

LEARNING TO SAY "NO!"

The emotional conflict that sometimes underlies chronic pain indicates that on some level we are afraid to claim our own thoughts and feelings in front of others. We are afraid to differ. The challenge of expressing ourselves is, of course, a challenge everyone faces. Learning personal authenticity is part of the journey of our lifetime. Not everyone experiences chronic pain in the process of learning personal authenticity. For some people, however, pain can act as a signal that we are sacrificing our personal truths too much to other people's needs and demands and that we need to change that pattern.

You can try numerous self-help techniques to identify the ultimate sources of your pain. You can also identify whether it would help you physically, as well as emotionally and spiritually, to strengthen your ability to own and express your feelings, including those that involve your differences from others. You can approach this task by looking at the quality of your relationships with other people.

SIGNS OF FEELING CONTROLLED

We can be bound to others both by love and affection and by negative feelings such as resentment, fear, and anger. When these negative feelings come up regularly, they indicate that in some way we feel controlled by another person. We feel disempowered, and this sense of disempowerment may be contributing to increased pain.

Typical signs of feeling disempowered include the sense that another person is repeatedly acting unjust and unkind, bossing us around too much, neglecting or hurting us, taking up our space, not taking on their share of the load, or demanding too much. In situations like these where we feel controlled, we may feel that no matter what we say, we aren't heard. In some cases, the way we address the situation can guarantee that our words won't have an adequate effect, and we disempower ourselves in the very act of speaking.

We may also feel that it is not safe for us to speak up and tell the other person what we feel. We may be afraid of speaking our minds, usually because of something learned in childhood. Today, these patterns may express themselves by our desire to avoid conflict. We think that if we speak up, the other person will react strongly to our words, yell at us, neglect us, or boss us around even more than usual. In the worst-case scenario, that person may hurt us physically. We may also think that by speaking our minds, we will hurt the other person's feelings too much. We may have learned to neglect our own feelings for the sake of taking care of other people. In these situations, we have strong blocks to speaking honestly.

Whatever the reason that we do not speak up, the result is that we harbor anger, fear, or resentment inside ourselves, a sure sign that we are creating self-destructive internal stress and that we need to speak up. We need to change the situation. If we don't, not only will we feel bad emotionally, but our negative emotions will eat away at us physically, enhancing the stress in our bodies by causing contraction and constriction and laying the foundation for chronic pain.

STRATEGIES FOR SAYING "NO!"

How can you identify when you need to speak up about something? If you are scared to speak up or feel it won't make any difference, what strategies can you use to help? Here are some ideas:

1. *Accept how you feel.* Sometimes we avoid speaking because we tell ourselves that we shouldn't feel the way we do. For example, let's say someone in your household is messy or loud. You tell yourself that you shouldn't be upset and that you should be able to handle this better. Or a friend gets on the phone and talks your ear off again and again about her problems. Even though you feel irritated, you tell yourself you shouldn't be short with her because she needs you. Let's say someone puts you down and your feelings are hurt. You tell yourself that it's your fault you're so sensitive! These are all ways of discounting how you feel and making your feelings unimportant. However, your feelings—including feelings of resentment, fear, or anger—are important. They are you, and they are making you sick! Whether or not you are correct in feeling the way you do is not the issue. The issue is to stop discounting your feelings and start accepting them. How you feel is how you feel. You *should* feel that way for no other reason than the fact that you do. Once you can acknowledge how you feel, you can begin to do something about it. First, however, you have to let what is going on inside you be okay because it is you.

2. *Vent your feelings.* As part of accepting how you feel, you will find a tremendous sense of relief and empowerment if you can vent those feelings full force. This is what Marilyn did. It is also what I did in the process of owning the validity of my feelings of anger and pain about my father's abandonment. Venting your feelings does not mean that you should vent them directly against the person with whom you are upset. After all, if you yell and scream at someone else, that person will only yell and scream back at you. But venting is important as part of your own personal process of owning your feelings—of letting it be okay to feel the way you feel. Vent your feelings in private. Roll up your car windows when you're driving, and yell out your frustrations. Take a walk and forcibly shout, "I won't take this anymore!" or "I won't let you control me!" When you are alone at home, beat the pillows on your bed or sofa and yell out to the person who is frustrating you just how you feel. The sheer power of your self-expression will help you convince yourself of the validity of how you feel and move you toward greater empowerment.

Just as venting your feelings is not about acting out on the person with whom you are upset, it also is not about complaining to a third party about a situation or a person. When you complain, you usually avoid empowering yourself. You avoid doing something to change the situation you are complaining about. You act as the victim.

Venting is about acknowledging to yourself how strongly you feel about an issue, instead of just repressing your feelings. By venting your feelings on your own, you will find a wonderful escape valve. You will also come to grips with how much your feelings matter to you and how powerful they really are. This will help you become clearer and more assertive when you do speak to others.

3. *Accept that there will be conflict in relationships.* When we have difficulty owning and expressing our feelings or stating our boundaries with others, this indicates a fear of conflict. Rather than confront the possibility of conflict, we shut up. Ironically, the more we avoid conflict, the more it is likely to burst out in a negative form: externally, in the form of heated arguments, upsets, yelling, or crying; internally, in the form of resentment, insecurity, and ill health. Creative conflict is an inherent aspect of healthy relationships. Creative conflict involves the ability to speak and hold your ground, even if your opinion differs from another's. It also involves the ability to hear others' points of view without fear or reaction and to negotiate differences of opinion.

You will know that you have a fear of creative conflict if you avoid speaking honestly to people in your life. The issue can be as small as the other person taking up too much of your time on the telephone, or as large as addressing concerns over a mate's fidelity. Ask yourself to whom you aren't speaking honestly and what you aren't saying. All the people in your life to whom you have trouble speaking control you. They may not intend to control you. Their intention is not the issue. The issue is how you react to their behavior. If you have difficulty speaking your mind, then you experience them as controlling, regardless of their intention. Therefore, you have to change yourself.

Make a list of the people you have difficulty speaking to honestly. Ask yourself what you are afraid of saying. What are you angry or resentful about? Once you are clear about who you feel controlled by and over what, you can begin to think about what you need to say.

Look at your fear of reprisals. When we don't speak up, we are usually afraid of reprisals or payback. We think that things will get worse if we speak up. Is this the case for you? What are you afraid will happen? Fear of reprisals keeps us locked up inside ourselves. Are you afraid that the other person will talk back? Or be mean? Or complain? None of these things can really hurt you that much. Facing your fear of reprisals is learning to stand up for yourself more effectively, and this is part of learning how to incorporate creative conflict into your relationships. It is also the key to reducing chronic pain.

If your fear involves a concern about being physically hurt—struck or beaten—then other forms of intervention may be necessary. Barring fear of physical injury, however, conquering your fear of the other person's reactions is part of learning to say, "I am your equal. My feelings count as much as yours. I want both to give and receive respect."

4. *Challenge your sense of obligation.* Whenever you feel you are doing something because you "should" do it, stop and ask yourself, "Do I really want to do this?" If you do, go ahead and give your whole heart to whatever you are doing. If you don't, see if you can step away and give yourself permission *not* to do what you think you should do, or to do it less often. Observe that the world does not collapse around you.

When you start questioning your need always to listen to the voice of obligation, others may well attack you for it. They may say, "But you are supposed to do this!" or "How could you not do that?" Be prepared to deal with such negative reactions. Consciously or unconsciously, others are utilizing an appeal to your sense of obligation to make you do something you may not want to do. They are also avoiding taking responsibility themselves by telling you to do something on the basis of social mores or some other authority rather than on the basis of their own feelings. Help them become conscious of their behavior with questions such as, "Why should I?" or comments such as "That may be how you feel, but it's not my view of the matter." Establish a new policy for yourself: you will be willing to listen to others with different points of view, but they should not try to persuade you to do anything out of obligation or guilt. If they can find a better and healthier motivation for you, maybe you'll change your mind. If not, you'll decide to do what you want.

If you feel confused about whether it is a sense of obligation or an innate sense of appropriateness or of desire that is guiding your choices, check in with your body. Your body will always tell you when you are making the wrong choices for yourself, including when you are considering the "shoulds" and "oughts" of your life. When we do what we "should" do and this conflicts with our deeper inner desire, the body gets tighter.

Years ago, when I had not yet sorted out my relationship with my rather needy mother, I began to notice that my neck periodically tightened during our conversations with each other. For example, if I was visiting her and got up to leave, and she asked me to stay a bit longer I would stay, but my neck would tighten in response to my decision. I was driven by obligation and guilt to stay a bit longer. I really wanted to leave but couldn't muster the courage to do so. I felt trapped and under stress, and my muscles reacted.

My mother was frequently depressed, and when she would start complaining about her life, I would try to soothe her, thinking that was the right thing to do. But my neck or chest would get tight. Eventually, I learned to confront my mother about her constant complaints, saying, for example, "Mommy, I love you, but are you aware that things go wrong for all of us in life? Complaining about things is burdensome for others, as well as for yourself!" I also learned to leave when I wanted to leave, rather than feeling I should stay because my mother asked me to. My neck and chest ceased to bother me when I was in my mother's company. I no longer felt trapped.

In the long run, listening to my own inner sense of what was right for me rather than to the harsh voice of duty helped me become more giving to my mother because I was less ambivalent. I knew that when I visited her, I really wanted to see her. She could feel the difference as well and began complaining less and appreciating me more.

A client of mine commented to me with surprise one day that he had just noticed a physical tension pattern that he had probably exhibited for years. This pattern told him a great deal about his relationship with his wife. He generally went to bed before she did, and took his time alone to read a book. One night, he realized that when he heard her come up the stairs, his entire body tensed. He knew she would want to talk to him and perhaps make some requests of him, at a time when he wanted peace and quiet. He realized that this tension response was a daily occurrence and that he had never told her what he wanted. Instead, acting like the nice husband he thought he should be, he listened to her and felt trapped. The feeling of being trapped by his sense of obligation was the tension in his body. To let go of it, all he had to do was to say, firmly and kindly, "Honey, I would love to talk to you some other time, but now is my quiet time. I'm sure you can understand." It was his sense of guilt that kept him from making a simple statement of what he needed.

Your body will always tell you whether you are following your sense of obligation and guilt or your own inner, organic sense of what is right for you. Listen to your body!

5. *Develop effective strategies for saying what you need to say.* Once you learn to accept and vent your feelings, challenge your sense of obligation and guilt, and recognize creative conflict as a healthy part of relationships, you need to develop effective strategies for communicating your point of view. If you have held back from owning your own truth with others, chances are that you need to build these strategies. Effective communication is a rare phenomenon, and it takes training to develop.

Let's say someone says or does something mean to you, so you yell back or complain. Do you notice how your behavior doesn't seem to change the situation? That person just ups the ante by yelling louder, putting you down, or ignoring you. You have used an ineffective strategy for speaking your mind.

To be effective, you have to speak from a place of authority and balance. You must state your feelings in a way that is calm, assertive, forceful, and respectful rather than emotional. Being calm has nothing to do with being cold or repressed. It is simply being free of stress-based reactions. Being free of emotional reactivity, even when talking about your emotions, compels the other person to listen to you, rather than just reacting. You will find that it is easier to find this calmer place of self-expression once you have fully vented your feelings. Then you will no longer need to explode, including at the person with whom you need to redefine boundaries!

Here are some tools for speaking out effectively.

a. Before speaking, think out what isn't working for you in the situation that bothers you. Then ask yourself how you can express this in a way that the other person might be able to hear. Can you express yourself without blame, while also being sure to assert your own boundaries? As an example, if a friend chews your ear off about her problems, can you tell her quietly and firmly, without emotional heat, that you appreciate that her life is difficult but that you also need support, or that you need more fun in your relationship? Alternatively, can you simply break into her complaints and calmly but clearly tell her that you appreciate her dilemmas, but unfortunately you have other things to attend to right now? Strategies such as these state your boundaries—in this case the fact that you need space—without attacking the other person.

b. Once you have thought out what you need to say, rehearse it through visualization. Do not simply talk through to yourself what you want to say. Role-play. *See and feel* yourself in the situation you envisage. By practicing how you will behave in a situation that is usually emotionally tense for you, you prepare yourself to let go of some of that tension. You rehearse being calm, clear, focused, and assertive: qualities that up to now you may have had trouble expressing with this person.

Visualization is a right-brain activity that has a profound capacity to retrain the way you react to situations. Visualization affects the neurological system directly. The brain's biochemistry does not distinguish between imagination and reality, so whatever we perceive programs our reactions. When we project in our imagination a new way of acting in a situation, that act of imagination begins to undermine old patterns of perception and behavior and to create the basis for new ones.

One of the first times I used visualization to change a behavior pattern of mine was during an earlier career as director of public affairs for a well-known college in New York City. I worked very closely with the president of the college, a man who tended to deal with his own insecurities by constantly criticizing his subordinates and questioning their decisions. Though I worked hard and successfully to improve the scope and efficiency of the office of public affairs, whatever I did was never enough. I used to come home from a twelve-hour day at work with my back hurting, feeling furious that my employer seemed to value so little of what I did. One night when I was obsessing over how to deal with him, I decided to begin to imagine how I wanted to be in his presence. I saw myself clear, relaxed, precise, confident, and assertive. In my imagination, I heard myself speaking calmly and forcefully and saw myself adopting an unhurried, relaxed demeanor. I not only *saw* myself as I wanted to look, I also *felt* myself as I wanted to feel. I envisaged feeling relaxed and at ease. My focus was on visualizing how *I* was going to be in the situation, not on how my employer was going to respond. Imagining how he was going to respond would have been closer to fantasy than to genuine visualization. In visualization, we use our mind to change ourselves, not others over whom we have no direct control. And through changing ourselves we change the environment around us.

In the course of my own visualization, I became increasingly peaceful and self-assured. The day after I visualized more empowering interactions with my employer, I began practicing what I had imagined while speaking with the president of the college. I kept at it, and slowly but surely, the president's attitude toward me altered. I had changed my own response pattern and was no longer being reactive to him. He responded by granting me greater respect.

When you practice visualization, begin by relaxing yourself through meditative breathing or a body scan. The imagination's creative power is stimulated by relaxation and inhibited by stress. The more relaxed you can be, the more effectively you will be able to visualize. Once you have released some of the tension from your body and mind, pick a situation in which you want to change your own response, to empower yourself more clearly, and to enable you to address the other person more effectively. As you imagine this situation, imagine how you want to *look*, what you want to *sound* like, and how you want to *feel*. You are rehearsing in your imagination how you want to be in a given situation before it happens. Then, while you are going through that actual situation, keep your visualization in mind so that it can strengthen your ability to replace stress-based, disempowering reactions with stronger, more confident ones. Observe the positive, concrete impact on your life of repeatedly utilizing your power of creative imagination in this way.

c. *Practice breath awareness and muscle relaxation in all situations that raise tension.* When you visualize, remember to include breath and body awareness in your practice, to help you identify what it feels like to respond proactively rather than defensively—to prevent a startle response—to situations in your life. Do the same thing in all interactions that provoke stress. Be present to your breathing in all potentially stressful situations. Practice breathing easily and deeply, and relax any muscle tension in your face, shoulders, or chest. You will be changing your physiological pattern, and this will result in a feeling of enhanced confidence and power.

Early in my career of teaching self-healing techniques for chronic pain, I would occasionally speak at conferences of traditionally oriented medical practitioners. While the medical community has become more open to alternative approaches, years ago this was not at all the case. I often encountered a crowd that was skeptical or downright hostile. It was important for me to focus on maintaining a calm center in my body through breath and body awareness and through consistently releasing any feelings of tension that I observed. This process enabled me to feel more grounded and clearer in my communications, to let go of anxiety, and to convey a sense of authority and knowledge to my audience. Similarly, your own practice of self-awareness through tuning in to your breath and to your muscles and paying attention to releasing tension will enhance your ability to stand your ground and to feel focused in any situation.

d. *Make eye contact.* When we are afraid, we tend to avoid eye contact. The other person reacts by failing to take us seriously or by suspecting that there is something devious or underhanded in our behavior. Make eye contact when you explain your feelings and state your boundaries. Hold the other person's attention. This may be difficult at first, but practice makes perfect.

e. *Repeat your strategies again and again.* Telling other people how you feel and asking for respect is not something you do only once. You have to be prepared to do it again and again. If you have had a habit of not telling others what you feel, you can't expect them to hear you clearly the first time around. Be prepared to express your feelings patiently and to state your needs many times over. Eventually, the other person will hear. In the process, you will overcome your fear, anger, and resentment. Your body will tell you how much better that feels.

6. *Become more proactive.* Learning to say "No!" to things that upset you—to let go of fear and anger by speaking up—is just one part of taking greater charge of your life. You can take even greater control, and feel more empowered, by going one step further: figure out more clearly what works for you, and plan how to get there. In addition to saying "No!" to what you don't want, actively say "Yes!" to what you do want. Become more proactive.

Being in pain makes us reactive as we become dependent on others. We need them to help us. The more we need others' help, however, the more we tend to let them define our lives. Unfortunately, this is not good for our health. Feelings of dependency encourage fear and anger because we give others the reins of control. Work on becoming more proactive. Think about what works for you, take responsibility for getting there, and see yourself as the control center of your life.

a. *Ask yourself how you can take greater control over the daily details of your life.* Look at your daily routine. Are there places where you wait for someone else to make the decisions for you? Where could you establish greater control? Rather than letting a family member, colleague, or friend decide what you are going to do, can you initiate decisions more? When it comes to your medical care, do you rely too much on your doctor's opinions? What do you need to do to make sure that you, and not another person, are making the decisions about your life?

b. *Strategize how to bring more of what you want into your life.* When you look at your life as a whole, what would give you a greater sense of pleasure and accomplishment? More friends? Greater involvement in the arts? More accomplishment or recognition at work or at home? A more regular exercise routine? Weight loss? Better nutrition? A spiritual practice? Taking those voice lessons you've been thinking about for years? Establish goals for yourself. Give yourself timelines for achieving them. Look at the weeks ahead, and outline where you want to be week by week. The more confidently you take responsibility for what you want and go after it aggressively, the more likely you are to feel less pain and more ease.

Vitality and health are strongly correlated with a sense of life purpose. That sense of purpose does not come automatically to most of us. But it can be learned. One of the best books for helping you deepen your understanding of, and commitment to, a sense of purpose in your life is Stephen R. Covey's *The 7*

Habits of Highly Effective People. It outlines specific strategies for changing reactive into proactive patterns and gaining greater control over the direction of your life. The result is often a reduction in chronic pain.

Life is difficult. This is a simple fact. We all have to deal with external obstacles, including many unanticipated and unwanted events. At the same time, we do create many of the opportunities and limitations of our own lives, both by our actions and by our neglect. Being increasingly proactive is the process by which we take greater responsibility for bringing what we want into our lives. This process is identical with the means by which we learn ever-greater personal empowerment. Expanding your personal sense of empowerment can reap enormous benefits in your ability to reduce chronic pain.

RECOMMENDATIONS

Learning to state your boundaries is an aspect of personal empowerment through which you can free yourself from negative emotions such as anger, resentment, anxiety, and fear and simultaneously reduce the physical pain and tension that accompany those negative emotions. Try to: (1) accept how you feel; (2) vent your feelings; (3) accept that there will be conflict in relationships; (4) challenge inappropriate or overbearing feelings of obligation; (5) develop effective communication strategies; (6) become more proactive. When you are more empowered, you are less susceptible to the emotional and physical stress that is the primary hallmark of feeling out of control of your life.

FURTHER READING

Stephen R. Covey, *The 7 Habits of Highly Effective People* (New York: Simon & Schuster, 1990). An excellent guide to the process of personal empowerment.

Roger Fisher and William Ury, *Getting to Yes: Negotiating Agreement Without Giving In* (New York: Penguin, 1983). A step-by-step strategy for win-win negotiations.

14

ROOTING OUT ATTITUDES THAT CREATE FEAR, ANGER, AND PAIN

Chronic stress is an inevitable outcome of any long-standing disempowerment. On a physiological level, that stress fosters neuromuscular tension, restricted breathing, and other fight-or-flight responses that contribute to chronic pain. Emotionally, feelings of disempowerment come out in chronic fear and anger. Chronic fear keeps us disempowered by making it difficult or impossible for us to take the initiative. Chronic anger reflects the fact that we cannot stand the situation we are in, but are afraid to change it. Regaining greater control over our lives and establishing proper boundaries for ourselves requires us to challenge the fear that holds us back, to vent our anger, and to adopt strategies to change the situation that is causing us stress. As we change the situation and set our own goals more proactively, the physiological signs of stress that are the corollaries of fear and anger subside and our chronic pain dissipates.

Whenever emotional stress triggers chronic pain, negative emotions of fear and anger become primary motivating factors in our behavior. Working on developing your ability to express yourself—your needs and boundaries—and developing your comfort level with your right to say "No" or to differ all contribute to reducing fear and anger, the stress they cause, and the pain that results from this stress. The inner signs that you are effectively reducing stress include being less driven by fear, suffering less anger, and being able to express your own opinions more forcefully and effectively. The outer signs of stress reduction include being able to resolve tensions in your life in a particular situation either by changing yourself or by changing or leaving the situation in question.

The challenge of reducing chronic emotional stress and physical pain includes identifying, confronting, and eliminating fear and anger as primary motivating forces in our lives. Sometimes meeting this challenge requires us to *root out deep attitudes and behavior patterns that inevitably either reflect fear and anger or serve to entrench these negative emotions in our lives.* We have already looked at how attitudes of obligation and guilt can have these effects. The following three case studies will show how other attitudes and behavior patterns can create chronic stress and how freeing yourself from these attitudes and behavior patterns will free you from chronic anger and fear.

JOANNE: PERFECTIONISM AND ANGER

Joanne was referred to me for treatment because of shoulder and neck pain, sometimes accompanied by headaches. An intelligent, thoughtful older woman, Joanne had been going through difficult times. Her husband had been ill for several years, and though he now seemed recovered, other problems had surfaced. Joanne's daughter had been diagnosed with cancer, and Joanne had had to cope with the shock and offer emotional and physical support. As a result, she had spent a great deal of time taking care of her daughter's three small children.

Joanne was exhausted. She was also disappointed and angry with her daughter, who seemed to lack any self-discipline, for not taking better care of herself. Why didn't she stop smoking? Why didn't she deal with her weight? If she couldn't take care of herself for her own sake, couldn't she at least do this for her children? She was leaving all the work and responsibility to Joanne, her mother!

Joanne was also angry with herself and felt guilty for being judgmental of her daughter. Joanne had been studying Buddhism and meditation for years and felt she should be past judging people by now. She was also upset with herself for not being more at peace with her life, for failing to find the inner calm that was her spiritual goal. In fact, Joanne seemed to be constantly angry with herself. She confessed that she even got angry with herself when she meditated. She chastised herself for being insufficiently spiritually developed if she didn't find perfect calm!

A perfectionist, Joanne drove herself and identified herself with her competency. She had to be able to fix everybody else's life. At the same time, she couldn't help resenting the demands her efforts to fix everyone else's were making on her own life. It was terribly draining. Joanne also had to be able to fix herself, and in her eyes, she needed lots of fixing! Even her aspirations to be a gentle, kind, spiritual person came with strings attached: the slightest failure in this regard was met with merciless self-criticism!

Joanne's feeling that she could never do anything right disempowered her. Her perfectionism was an internal reflection of a harsh superego. Joanne's perfectionism also guaranteed frustration, as she could not possibly meet her own standards. The result: more anger at herself.

Joanne's chronic anger fed her neck and shoulder tension and gave her headaches. To get rid of her chronic pain, Joanne had to stop demanding perfection. She had to stop the habit of letting anger at herself motivate her behavior—whether that behavior involved doing more for her daughter or criticizing herself for spiritually imperfect behavior.

Joanne worked on letting go of her perfectionism by letting go of responsibility for her daughter. Though she continued to help her, she pulled back whenever she noticed feelings of resentment or anger against her daughter surfacing. Joanne also worked on letting go of trying to whip herself into spiritual shape. When she noticed that she was angry, rather than criticizing herself for this and intensifying her anger, she tried to notice and accept. She worked on living by the principle that self-acceptance, not competency, is the road to greater inner peace. She gave up on competency, including spiritual competency, for the sake of peace. Her anger decreased, since that anger was fueled by the need to be perfect, and her headaches and upper body pain gradually eased.

Joanne improved her physical health by working on letting go of anger and of the perfectionism that reflected and motivated that anger. In the process, she changed her situation and herself. She changed her situation by giving her daughter greater responsibility over her own life, rather than trying to fix things for her. She changed herself by learning to guide her behavior through self-acceptance rather than self-criticism.

DIANE: NEEDINESS AND FEAR OF ABANDONMENT

Diane's story is an interesting study in chronic pain that seemed to have a purely physical origin but that ended up being intimately linked to emotional issues. Diane came to me with severe physical pain in her right arm and shoulder. The pain was the result of an accident six months earlier. Diane had injured her right hand, including almost severing one finger, when she had mistakenly put her hand through a window. Surgery had left one nerve dead, and she had gone through months of physical therapy. Though the surface wound had healed, the pain in her arm and shoulder had increased. After some treatment, she had been told that she had neuropathy, a chronic nerve pain that allopathic medicine sometimes finds difficult to treat. Doctors had told her that her condition unfortunately would no doubt worsen.

Diane was going through a difficult time in her life. At forty-three, she was a manager in a large hotel chain, something that created a fair amount of stress. She was also in the process of working out the final details of a divorce, which was emotionally and monetarily difficult, especially since she had taken on extra financial burdens in order to obtain sole custody of her two young sons.

Diane had had her first child at the age of twenty-six after a problematic pregnancy and extremely long and difficult labor. The early months of nursing had also been sleepless. Diane had gradually come to the realization that her husband was completely unavailable for helping with the family. Despite this, when she accidentally became pregnant again six years later, she decided to have another child. The birth of a second child led to no improvement in her relationship with her husband. Factors other than her husband's lack of responsibility toward the children also indicated that the relationship was unhealthy. For example, between the birth of her first and second children, Diane had been in a car accident that had totaled her car and injured her. Her husband had blamed her for the accident and had been unsupportive throughout her recuperation.

Diane had injured her hand at a symbolically crucial moment, on a day shortly after she had initiated the divorce proceedings. She had decided for the sake of the children to invite her husband's parents over for dinner. In the course of the evening, she had gone to open a window and had instead pushed her hand right through the window and had had to be hospitalized.

As Diane told me the details of her life, her eyes filled with tears. I encouraged her to feel her pain and, after a few minutes, asked her if she could articulate what it was about. She became quiet and then said, "I still love my husband. I know he has behaved terribly toward me again and again, but I feel that we have a soul's connection, a deep love."

Right there, Diane unwittingly revealed what we later came to realize was one of the causes of the escalating physical pain in her right arm. It was not love that Diane felt. She had an addiction to unfulfilled emotional longing that she unconsciously associated with intimacy. She assumed that relationship required pain, and so she clung to pain. Diane had stayed in an unloving relationship for many years, learning to ask for little, even as she kept on convincing herself that there might be something there. She was still emotionally committed to the pain of this relationship, even though she was going through a divorce. Under these conditions, how could her body *not* suffer?

Diane was clinging to a relationship that left her constantly abandoned, needy, and in a state of emotional collapse. What Diane interpreted as love was actually a relationship of dependency in which, whenever she was hurt, instead of working to establish better boundaries for herself and to reevaluate her feelings toward her husband, she held on to her perceived need for him. Consequently, she also held on to the hurt, even through divorce. Then, because she couldn't move through or resolve her hurt since she was attached to what was causing her emotional pain, she expressed that pain somatically.

Interestingly enough, the injury to her hand was not the first time Diane had unconsciously resorted to physical self-mutilation to enact the psychic pain of her self-destructive and personally disempowering attachments. It was no accident that she had been in a car accident between her two pregnancies. And she had spent a surprising amount of her life recovering from accidents. Prior to her involvement with her husband, she had been in two serious accidents, one of which had resulted in her being hospitalized for months. Both accidents had occurred immediately subsequent to an interaction with her mother in which her mother had abandoned her emotionally. In both cases, instead of fighting for her rights or expressing her feelings strongly, Diane had kept her feelings to herself and had immediately gotten into an accident that externally mirrored her internal trauma. The events of her life symbolically portrayed the psychic mutilation that she felt from the people to whom she was attached. She stayed in attachments that disempowered her, feeling needy and abandoned and at the same time unable to ask for more.

Diane wasn't going to get over her attachment to pain unless she took a clear look at the behavior patterns of the people she felt she needed in her life and asked herself if she were getting an equal return. Where she was not, she had to demand her rights or leave. Even though she was a capable career woman, Diane needed to develop emotional autonomy.

In one of our early sessions, I asked Diane if, given how her husband had behaved toward her, a stronger attitude might not be more appropriate—something like "I don't want you anywhere near me!" or "Get out of my life!" Diane recognized that she really was very angry. She was then able to own her feeling of anger and become more empowered, rather than acting out her self-imposed disempowerment through physical suffering. During this session, the pain in her arm diminished markedly. Encouraged by this result, Diane went home and worked on being inwardly clearer and more decisive about wanting to let go of a relationship that had not been healthy for her. She could stand on her own two feet and be proud of it!

Diane and I worked together many times on specific instances in her life that had involved her tendency to be needy, to feel she couldn't afford to ask for more, and to feel dependent on others for whatever she could get. In all of these situations, the disempowering attitude that expressed Diane's default position was "I can't express my needs more strongly, or they will abandon me." She had felt she couldn't express her needs with her husband, but this had turned out to be far from an isolated pattern. For example, she felt she couldn't confront her child care person, who abused the privileges she gave her, lest the girl stop working for her altogether. Similarly, even though she was close to the top of the heap in the world of hotel management, she felt she couldn't tell her employer that it was important for her to be able to take a ten-day vacation. Her heavy responsibilities and status certainly entitled her to as much!

In each case, when Diane risked asking for more, she got it. She worked on moving from neediness and collapse to independence, and on modeling greater assertiveness, freedom, and power in her interactions with other people.

Diane made very rapid progress in healing from a neurological problem that doctors had said would only get worse with time. Within three months, her neuropathy was virtually gone. In the six years since that time, it has not returned. Diane's progress was due primarily to the fact that she was completely open to interpreting her physical pain as an expression of emotional crisis. She looked deeply at the emotional issues that our sessions raised and moved to change herself in significant ways. She wanted to heal physically, but she also wanted to heal emotionally, to develop greater personal autonomy and balance.

Diane worked to let go of her deep fear of abandonment. In the process, she changed herself by changing her fundamental emotional motivations, shifting from fear to greater confidence. She changed her situation with her husband, her employer, and her child care person. And in one case, the case of her dysfunctional relationship with her husband, she left the situation that was disempowering her by finalizing her divorce and leaving him.

KRISTIN: VICTIM CONSCIOUSNESS, RESENTMENT, AND FEAR

Kristin came to me with complaints of severe chronic fatigue and fibromyalgia, which had forced her to resign two years before from a job in the corporate world in which she had been in charge of investor relations for a powerful investment brokerage firm. Thirty-eight years old, Kristin had been successful but unhappy in her work. She had never felt adequately recognized in what she viewed as a macho world and hadn't liked the work she was doing. She had been resentful of her situation but fearful of taking responsibility for quitting and seeking alternative employment. Now her forced resignation due to illness had given her an opportunity to rebuild her life along lines that suited her better. She was training to be a massage therapist.

Unfortunately, even though Kristin now said she wanted to be a massage therapist, she also continued to bring the ambivalent dynamics that had plagued her in her corporate career into this new arena. She alternated between being interested in the work, on the one hand, and feeling that she was being forced by financial need to pursue her training and establish a new career, on the other. When she adopted the latter perspective, instead of looking forward to her future, she lived in dread of trying to make it on her own. Feeling this way is normal for anyone in transition, but you also have to move through and override this state in order to be successful. If not, you act the victim by letting what seem to be external circumstances control you, rather than taking control of your own life. You disempower yourself and then blame life for your situation.

Kristin spent a disproportionate amount of time in anxiety and dread. She was afraid of the independence she also wanted and fearful of asserting herself, and she lacked skills for doing that. Her illness both expressed the stress she was under and gave her permission to act out an unconscious motivation: play the victim, avoid responsibility, and stay stuck. She could always say she was too sick to move forward.

Kristin's father had been a drifter, setting a poor example of self-motivation. Her mother had been nonsupportive and critical. Kristin had learned from her mother's critical attitudes that it was pointless to share her own opinions. When children have this experience, some react by trying to be supergood and others become outwardly rebellious. Kristin had chosen a different route: withdrawal. As a child, Kristin had frequently retreated to her room, saying to herself that there was no point in doing what her parents wanted, because whatever she did, it was never enough. She often found her way to the one thing that she knew she could do to feel safe: she slept.

As an adult, Kristin still did the one thing she could do to feel safe: she slept. She developed chronic fatigue syndrome. To get better, one of the things Kristin had to do was to learn not to be a victim. In her case, this meant not relying on illness as a vehicle for avoiding making choices in her life, whether that choice involved showing up at a therapy session, attending a training class in her profession of choice, making a business plan, hammering out a financial arrangement with a new client, taking responsibility for her diet and health, or developing a strategy for getting better over time.

Every time Kristin felt she couldn't do something because she felt ill, we considered the possibility that it might be an unconscious way to avoid making decisions over her life. We made a contract. According to this contract, each week she was to take initiatives despite feeling poorly, and despite her anxiety and dread. The initiatives ranged in size and significance. Some involved slowly building up her exercise regimen, whether or not she felt like exercising and even when she felt she didn't have the strength. Some involved being consistent in coming to her meetings with me. Some involved overcoming anxiety and dread by making business plans and committing to deadlines in her professional development. In all of these cases, Kristin painstakingly began to challenge the anxiety that made her want to withdraw. She slowly began to develop a little more trust in her ability to direct herself in her career and her life, rather than seeing her life as out of her control in a world in which everything just seemed to happen to her.

Kristin stayed stuck—and ill—as long as she held on to resentment, to the disempowering assumption that somehow someone or something else was controlling her life. Once she decided, painfully and slowly, to try to move forward regardless of how she felt physically, the severity of her illness dissipated. Kristin worked on letting go of a disempowering attitude that someone or something else was always to blame for her life. Anxiety was the driving force behind that attitude, so Kristin worked on confronting and dealing with the negative emotion of anxiety. In the process, she developed more autonomy. Kristin changed her life by changing herself. Her changed attitude toward herself helped her to deal more effectively with the situation she was in and to begin to overcome some of her own limitations.

HEALING YOURSELF OF NEGATIVE EMOTIONS

When long-term pain signals that we feel disempowered in our lives, we live in the startle reflex mode, unable to feel safe or satisfied. Something is controlling us. What that something is may feel as if it is external, as in the case of Kristin, who felt controlled first by her employers and then by her illness. Alternatively, the controlling force that disempowers us may feel as if it is internal, as in the case of Joanne, whose negative self-criticism constantly cut her down. Healing involves empowering ourselves, which involves identifying and letting go of the dynamics that keep us disempowered. The three stories of Joanne, Diane, and Kristin help identify four strategies for regaining empowerment and improving health.

1. Consider your motivations, and replace anger or fear with the value of inner balance. We rarely consider the deeper motivations of our behavior. Unfortunately, negative emotions such as fear and anger often play a role in those motivations. Of the two emotions, fear is the more basic one, and it can deeply color our most basic life choices. My first book, *The Art of Effortless Living*, focuses on the process by which we can learn to replace fear with more self-affirming values. In that book, I describe a meeting I had with a very successful tort lawyer whose fear-based behavior was completely camouflaged by his rationalizations about life. We met at a dinner party. He was interesting and, at a point in our conversation, began telling me how worried he was for his seventeen-year-old son. He thought his son, who was quite gifted, was not sufficiently realistic and therefore was likely to be hurt by the real world. The son didn't want to go to the college his father recommended because he found the competitive environment too cutthroat. Instead, he had chosen for himself an institution that focused on a more collaborative approach to learning but that the father felt was less prestigious. This son was also an exceptional sportsman and team player. He took pleasure in speaking with members of the opposing team after games and treated them as people with a common interest stemming from their love of sports. He was critical of the hostile approach that often pitted opposing team members against one another and that sometimes led to fights. The father admired his son's attitude but also told me, "My son is going to get hurt because he thinks too highly of people." Instead of encouraging his son's behavior as setting an example for others, he fretted and actively discouraged his son from becoming a model for others because he found his son's behavior naive and unrealistic.

When the conversation turned to this man's professional work as a tort lawyer, he said he didn't in principle approve of hostile, competitive approaches but had no problem with this at work because as a lawyer, if he didn't thrash his opponent, his opponent would thrash him. He also told a story about some investment bankers who had come to him for advice on whether or not to invest millions of dollars in the tobacco industry. The lawyers were concerned that recent legal actions taken by the U.S. states against tobacco companies would hurt the profitability of their investments. The lawyer I was speaking with was not himself a smoker and said that he personally felt smoking was bad for one's health, but he found it perfectly acceptable to deal with this situation from a purely financial perspective. He ended up strongly recommending to the wealthy investors that they continue to put their money into the tobacco industry.

This man was well intentioned. He loved his wife and children and worked hard. But he was deeply enmeshed in living in a way that justified doing things that another part of him felt were not acceptable. He loved his son's courage and idealism but sought to discourage them as unrealistic. He felt that aggression and hostility were bad but rationalized his own competitive ethic as a lawyer by saying the profession made him act that way. He knew smoking was destructive to health, including the health of his own children and future generations but recommended investing in the tobacco industry. Like so many people, he had built a financially and socially successful life while sacrificing his inner values on the grounds that he couldn't survive if he lived according to his ideals.

This man was subtly addicted to fear. He rationalized his life decisions by saying that he could not do otherwise. And why could he not do otherwise? Because of what "other people" did, because of the "demands of his profession," or because that was just "the way life is." He excused his own inability to stand for what inwardly he felt was right by saying that something or someone else—other people, society, or human nature—was forcing him to behave the way he behaved. He was disempowered. I was not surprised to find, toward the end of our evening together, that he had developed serious joint pain.

At some level, the tort lawyer's story is everybody's story. We all have to struggle with letting go of fear and of the anger that usually accompanies fear. We all have to find our way to embodying what feels right for us, despite the obstacles society presents and despite what others may think. The challenge is to make the process of letting go of fear conscious, to embrace it, and to commit to values of inner balance that replace fear.

Each of the four characters described above had to challenge his or her fear and anger. Joanne did it most consciously: she decided not to react to her own tendency to get angry with herself. She began to value being peaceful over being angry, so that when she noticed herself being angry either with herself or with others, she backed away from what she was doing, so as to establish greater inner balance. She decided not to feed her anger and to let go of allowing anger to be her motivating force. Diane challenged her fear of abandonment over and over again. She dared to ask for equal treatment and to let go of people who would not treat her with respect. Kristin learned to challenge her fear as well. She gradually let go of giving herself excuses, most particularly the excuse of her illness, to avoid making choices in her life.

Ask yourself where fear or anger motivates your behavior. Ask yourself what would be required of you to let go of some of that fear or anger. Are you willing to challenge any habit you may have of living with negative emotions?

2. *Commit yourself to greater autonomy.* Letting go of fear and anger means making a commitment to greater autonomy, to the ability to be self-reliant and self-determining. We all face disempowering situations. In my own process of healing from chronic pain, I had to learn greater autonomy in three different areas: I needed to learn to own my own feelings, whether or not others agreed with me; I needed to develop and define a unique career path as part of my own quest for myself; and I needed to develop financial autonomy, to free myself from economic dependency on others and to give myself the secure material base that would enable me to be whom I needed to be. Your challenges to developing personal autonomy are no doubt different from mine. We each have a unique path. Yet there is no question that the capacity for independence, even in the midst of our connections to others, is an important ingredient in reducing stress and maintaining or regaining health. It is also inherently satisfying. The more we can nurture ourselves, the safer we feel.

Are there any areas in which you need to develop a greater sense of autonomy? Describe these to yourself. What steps can you take to increase your independence? Develop a strategy that you can implement over the next six months to a year.

3. *When disempowerment strikes, change yourself, change the situation, or leave the situation.* Feelings of disempowerment always carry a price tag. That tag is the persistence of a negative emotion that seems to dictate your behavior. While the dominant negative emotions are fear and anger, there are many variations on this theme: resentment, frustration, irritation, jealousy, envy, anxiety, and panic are some. The persistence of a negative emotion is nature's call to action. That emotion tells you that something has to change in order for you to feel empowered. Look at any situation you are in that creates chronic tension or negative feelings, and consider how to change it.

Change can happen from one or more of three directions. First, you can change yourself by changing your attitude toward a situation. For example, if I feel constantly hurt by someone else's behavior, I can decide to change my attitude. I can decide that I don't care, not out of defense—which is another form of disempowerment—but after taking a good long look at a situation and seeing if I am getting what I want. Diane changed her attitude about her husband, deciding that she really didn't love him. This helped her view his behavior with detachment, and not to be affected by it.

Second, you can change the situation. Let's say that you have a family member who tends to drown you out whenever you get into a conversation. Let's say that your habit has been to shut up and fume or else to yell at that person, neither of which is very constructive. Perhaps you can change the situation by calmly, forcefully, and repeatedly stating that you are not available for one-way monologues. Alternatively, you can tell the person that you will talk with him when he is willing to listen to you. You thus take charge and alter the dynamics in a way that respects your boundaries.

As a third option, you can leave the situation. If the other person never stops yelling or dominating the conversation, you can simply decide to leave. If a relationship or a job doesn't work for you, after trying other options, perhaps your best decision is to walk out.

Make a list of situations in your life that create negative feelings of fear, anger, irritation, hurt, or jealousy. What are you willing to do to resolve your feelings of disempowerment? Where can you change yourself? Is this appropriate? How can you change the situation, to fit your own needs better? Do you need to leave the situation? Feeling empowered is about taking the initiative. Creating change is also about taking the initiative. Be willing to make change in your life.

RECOMMENDATIONS

Chronic fear and anger are negative emotions that carry a price tag of stress, tension, and pain. When our behavior is motivated by fear and anger or when attitudes that we have engender fear and anger in us, we are likely to suffer physically. The stories of Joanne, Diane, and Kristin exemplify three types of attitudes that express and foster fear and anger and can contribute to chronic pain: perfectionism, neediness, and playing the victim. Healing from the stress and disempowerment associated with such attitudes requires making personal balance, autonomy, and self-sufficiency our most important values. Strategically, this means we must be willing to risk change for the sake of pursuing these values and to let go of disempowering attitudes. Fear, disempowerment, and physical pain go together. Empowerment, physical health, and freedom from fear also go together.

FURTHER READING

Caroline Myss, *Sacred Contracts* (New York: Harmony Books, 2001). An exploration by a medical intuitive of how to become conscious of the unconscious contracts we make with life and how to let go of disempowering contracts and embrace empowering ones.

15

CONQUERING YOUR FEAR OF
PHYSICAL PAIN

One form of fear is unique to people who suffer from chronic pain, and that is fear of pain. You wake up in the morning, and as you roll over to get out of bed, your back spasms, or you feel a jabbing sensation in your shoulders or neck, or your hip complains. You get up from your chair to walk across the room and feel a sharp pain in your bad knee, or your head throbs, or your feet ache. If you didn't start to worry earlier, you do now. You ask yourself, "Will the pain get worse?" "Is it going to be there all day?" "Am I going to be able to do the things I had planned on getting done?" What about that walk you were going to take with a friend? Or the dinner at a nice restaurant?

As you think these thoughts, you anticipate and worry about pain that hasn't yet occurred. This is a natural tendency. After all, pain is worrisome. The problem, however, is that worry and anxiety increase the likelihood that you will feel pain because they increase the level of tension in your body. Your fear of pain makes pain more likely because it creates stress.

The medical system sometimes inadvertently stimulates our fear of pain, keeping us moving from doctor's visit to doctor's visit. If we go to a doctor for a chronic pain pattern and are told that the cause is something structural over which we have no control, it automatically triggers a sense of fear. Then when we feel pain, because we think we can do nothing about it, we feel more fear. The fear creates stress, which aggravates the pain, which eventually leads us back to the doctor. We perceive the doctor as our sole resource in the battle over something over which we have no control—our pain—and which presumably has a cause independent of us. We are disempowered! Feelings of lack of control trigger fear, which in turn triggers increased pain, which triggers another visit to the doctor, who finds another reason for our pain that is beyond our control, and so on. By causing us to see ourselves as helpless, the medical model intensifies our fear. Our fear intensifies our pain, and we become victims of chronic pain.

In order to eliminate your pain, you must conquer your fear of pain. How can you fight against the natural yet self-defeating tendency to worry about pain? Four tools can help you mobilize the power to free yourself of your fear of physical pain: visualization, breath awareness, developing a loving relationship with your body, and mobilizing your psychological strength. The use of each of these techniques will not only help you manage your fear of pain; it will also reduce your pain and improve your physical health.

VISUALIZATION

When you worry, you visualize a negative future outcome. You imagine that something bad is going to happen. This negative visualization has a neurological and muscular effect that contracts your muscles. This often brings about the very pain that you fear most. Chances are, your negative image of the future—your fear that your back won't hold up during dinner or that you will have a headache all day—causes you to contract the most in your weak points, the specific areas where you tend to feel pain. Your worry thus becomes a self-fulfilling prophecy.

To maneuver your way out of becoming an unwitting coconspirator in creating your own pain, you have to use the power of imagination to visualize positive rather than negative outcomes. If you do this, not only do you undo the effect of negative thinking and encourage your body to stay relaxed, you also send neurological messages that encourage a healing response.

Much of visualization is unconscious. We experience this all the time when we worry about something bad happening and . . . it happens! Even though, in these situations, we may tell ourselves that we don't want the thing we fear to happen, unconsciously we contribute to what we fear through the visual projections that are part of our worry. Let's say you worry by unconsciously visualizing that you will feel pain when you get out of a chair or go for a walk. Because your negative thought and image encourage your muscles to contract, you do in fact feel pain when you get up or walk. Then your mind tells you that you were justified in worrying because what you feared in fact happened! You are in a vicious cycle of fear creating pain, which creates more fear, which creates more pain. If instead you consciously visualize your body feeling and looking strong when you get out of your chair or take a walk, you might feel better. This takes some practice, but it is well worth the effort.

I first discovered both the power of positive visualization for healing my body and the negative influence that unconscious and habitual visualizations were exerting, totally by chance. At that time, my back bothered me on a daily basis. Every time I stood up from a chair I hurt, and I had to pause to loosen up before going into motion. I was discouraged and tired of the pain.

On this particular day, I was sitting in my armchair, and I began daydreaming wistfully about the actress Audrey Hepburn. For me, Audrey Hepburn has always been the epitome of grace and lightness. In my imagination, I saw that beautiful, angelic creature sitting on a chair with her eager childlike body and radiant smile. She was so graceful—and so unlike me! Then I imagined her rising effortlessly out of her chair, and as she did so, something impelled me to rise out of my own chair—*painlessly!* I was shocked. It was the first time in months that I had stood up free of pain. What had happened? I had to try this again.

I sat down in my chair again, imagined Audrey Hepburn sitting in her chair, and at the very moment that I imagined her rising in her inimitably light and gracious manner, I too rose. This time, however, my back hurt. So I experimented some more. As I experimented, I began to realize that the times I got up painlessly were the times when I was totally involved in the image of Audrey Hepburn and forgot about myself. The times when I experienced pain, my visualization was not so strong, and I held some element of doubt in my mind.

I had just discovered that focusing *intensely* on an image of how you want to be can produce astonishing effects. I started pretending to be Audrey Hepburn at every opportunity I could find. I knew I couldn't do this tentatively if I wanted to get results. I had to do it all the way. I really had to be Audrey Hepburn in my mind.

My experiments taught me that the more vividly and continuously I kept the image of Audrey Hepburn in my mind, the more it would help me. It wasn't enough to use that image once or twice, or even to spend just fifteen minutes a day using her image to influence my own bodily patterns. After all, I needed to replace images that I had held unconsciously and constantly for a number of years, images that committed me to pain. I had unwittingly cherished a vision of myself as incapacitated. Visualization was teaching me this and teaching me how to change my self-destructive habit.

I also started experimenting with other body visualizations. I bought videotapes of yoga teachers, movement specialists, athletes, and dancers, all people who moved powerfully, freely, and gracefully. I watched the tapes, absorbing the movements and imagining what it must feel like to be those people. I held in my own mind an image of a dancer moving when I walked down the street or went from room to room in my house. I imagined feeling and looking as that dancer must feel and look. I saturated myself with the visual and physical feel of strong, limber, graceful people. I was working on overriding the familiar visual program that I had unconsciously held in my mind for years. That program identified my body with restriction, limitation, and pain. By changing my program, I changed my body.

Our imaginations affect our physiology and biology far more profoundly than any act of conscious will. Imagination can bring a powerful new dimension of healing into your life. Images you hold in your mind can teach your body not only how to let go of fear-based programs but also how to move effectively in a way that you could never teach yourself consciously. Your unconscious mind takes your visualizations of free and healthy movement and transforms them into physiological, neurological, and biochemical input that reduces your pain. Try this: create the image of how you want to be in your mind, then let your brain do the work of bringing your body into line.

In order to practice seeing your body functioning well and to get the full benefit of your visualizations, you will have to fight the tendency to want to worry. However, the more you do this, the better your body is likely to feel.

How can you use positive visualization? First, you can use it for rehearsal. If you tend to think you will feel pain when you climb out of bed, then in your imagination see and feel yourself looking and feeling relaxed, limber, and comfortable *before* you actually do so. Take the time to immerse yourself thoroughly in your visualization. Then, once you have thoroughly rehearsed, engage in the action that has caused you to worry, and observe the results.

Rehearsal builds confidence and relaxation. You can rehearse how you want to feel and move at any time of the day and anywhere from a few minutes a day to repeatedly throughout the day.

Visual rehearsal begins to retrain your body's unconscious, automatic programs. To get optimum results out of your visualization, however, you should combine rehearsal with using visualization *simultaneously* with doing the thing that causes you fear. For example, if you are concerned about your ability to walk without a painful limp, you should not only rehearse seeing and feeling yourself walking easily *before* you walk, you should also imagine feeling and looking pain-free *while* you are taking your walk. Even if you feel pain, continue using the visualization. This will trigger a reaction in your body that will counteract the tendency to move in a way that produces pain. You may not feel completely free of pain, but chances are that if you stay with your visualization, you will feel less pain than otherwise. Over days, weeks, and months, your regular visualization will continue to improve your body mechanics.

Eventually, positive visualization will become not only a tool that you use on occasion but the way you look at your life and your body all the time—with positive rather than negative anticipation. You are practicing mind-body medicine, which will slowly but surely retrain your body's response patterns.

If you are new to visualization or feel you need to develop your visualization skills, I have developed a program on audiocassette or CD that can be ordered through my Web site or by using the order form at the end of this book.

FOCUS ON YOUR BREATHING

If you find yourself worrying about pain, move your attention away from your fear and focus instead on your breathing. Distract yourself. Bring all your awareness into the feeling of the breath, encouraging it to open and soften.

Worry and fear are addictive. They can act as a form of magical thinking, or attempt to control. This does not mean that we consciously think that by worrying about something, we will make it better. Rather, on some level we fear that if we let go of our worry, something bad will happen! If you have a digestive disorder, though it may help you to do something concrete to help it, it certainly doesn't help you to worry about it. Similarly, if you have back pain, it doesn't help you to worry about it. And yet not only do we worry, we may even think it's foolish *not* to worry! As if not worrying were on some level being irresponsible! Yet this is far from the case, since worry and fear only aggravate pain.

By focusing on your breathing when you are afraid of pain, you train yourself to defuse the worry response and, along with that, the stress and muscular contraction that worry brings in its train. You also automatically relax your entire body, since breath awareness promotes neuromuscular relaxation. You pull yourself out of the vicious pain/fear cycle. I have watched many people turn what could have become a major physical trauma into a passing minor event simply by focusing on their breathing to guide themselves through the pain without reacting to it.

The very last experience I had of crippling pain resolved itself for me primarily through use of the breath. I had pulled a muscle in a fast-moving yoga class, and twenty-four hours later my midback suddenly went into an agonizing spasm. Before I knew it, I was down on the floor, groaning and sobbing. I was terrified. It had been a very long time since I had felt such intense pain. Crying, I crept to my bed. As the night came on, visions of my past repeating itself swept before me. Did this pain mean I would be out of commission for long periods of time again? Had my body decided to collapse, just as unpredictably as it had done years before, and with such devastating results? The more my mind raced through its worries, the worse the pain became.

Somehow I got hold of myself. I began to breathe. I felt as though I were in a battle with my own inner demons, and I was. I had to calm my fears, or I was through. I knew that if I couldn't calm myself, my body could spiral down a vicious cycle. And so, all night long, I breathed. I drew my attention away from the pain and breathed. I trusted that with the focus on the breath, everything would be okay.

The next morning, I breathed as I got out of bed, breathed as I prepared breakfast, and breathed as I started my workday. The pain was still there, but it was much, much quieter. I kept on breathing, especially whenever fear began to overtake me. Three days later, the pain was gone. The experience taught me a painful lesson: years before, when I had suffered so much and for so long, a major factor in my pain had been my fear of pain. My fear had wound the tourniquet of pain ever tighter around my body. This time, by focusing on my breathing, I released that tourniquet and gave my body a chance to heal.

DEVELOP A LOVING RELATIONSHIP WITH YOUR BODY

When we worry about our body, we foster a negative attitude toward it and toward the sensations it harbors. We feel a jab of pain and worry that there will be another. We fear our sensations. We feel that our body is failing us. Our body becomes our enemy. Well, you can be sure that the body is aware of that and that such an attitude constitutes quite a stress for you. Your body is you!

You can help your body to feel better by not putting it into the role of the enemy. How can you do this? Earlier chapters discussed how important it is simply to observe, accept, and avoid judgment about your sensations, whether those sensations involve your breathing, your muscles, or your feelings of pain. Avoiding judgment is a form of love. For example, being nonjudgmental with friends—listening to them and accepting wherever they are at the moment, without criticism or advice—expresses love. Your friends feel this and open up. Similarly, if friends or family members are nonjudgmental and accepting with you, you no doubt feel loved, and you relax and feel better.

Apply loving nonjudgment to your body. Treat it like a dear friend. Accept your sensations, including your pain, without evaluating them. Assume that your body can find its own way to feeling better. See if over time you can replace negative reactions to your body—"Oh no, it hurts, is it going to hurt more?" or "I hate the way my body feels"—with acceptance—"Hmm. There is another sensation. How interesting. Let me just absorb that and see where it goes." Letting go of your fear about your body and replacing it with faith is likely to reward you with a reduction in pain.

A vivid experience taught me unequivocal trust in the power of loving, nonjudgmental presence to your body. I had been to a dinner party for the evening. I went to bed feeling fine but woke up at two in the morning with terrible stomach cramps, probably from food poisoning. I went to the bathroom and tried to vomit, but that didn't seem to help. I lay doubled over in bed, overwhelmed by my cramps. Usually, when we are in pain, something inside us also resists and fights the pain. And so as I lay there fighting my pain, a small voice came into my head, saying, "You always talk about nonjudgmental presence. Practice it now! Appreciate how you feel, no matter what that's like!" I listened. I focused on the sensations of pain in my intestines. I allowed them to be whatever they wanted to be. And then something remarkable happened.

At first the pain intensified, to the point where I felt I could not bear it any longer. Then, all of a sudden, I felt a rush of energy move through my body, from my abdomen to my head and then out of my head, leaving me crying with relief. The pain was completely gone! I was stunned. How had the abdominal cramps vanished?

From a medical perspective, what happened to me might seem inexplicable, but I believe that what occurred was quite simple. As I observed my sensations of pain without judgment, I allowed the tissues involved to relax. As they relaxed, the tension and pressure of the pain found a natural pathway to release itself. That pathway happened to be up through the connective tissue of my torso. With the tension released, the pain disappeared. Ever since that experience, I have many times used nonjudgmental appreciation of my sensations of pain to help them find a natural, organic pathway for release.

MOBILIZE YOUR PSYCHOLOGICAL STRENGTH

Refusing to dwell on negative experiences is an important part of lessening their effect. This applies not only to negative emotional experiences—for example, when someone criticizes you in a hostile, rejecting manner—but also to the negative experience of pain. Fighting the tendency to let pain take you over, depress you, or make you feel defeated has positive physiological as well as psychological benefits. You counter the fear response that causes muscle contraction, assert your power over your life, and bring into your body more of the energy that it needs to heal. You feel empowered. Feelings of empowerment always have a healthy effect.

Kristin (see page 206) took on the challenge of mobilizing her psychological strength by repeatedly doing things that she thought she couldn't do because of her illness. When she was afraid she wouldn't be able to make an appointment, she would challenge herself to make it. When she wanted to collapse into bed and pull the covers over her head, she told herself to wait just an hour longer before she did so. In some cases, this might not be the right approach, but for Kristin, whose fear of illness paralyzed her, it was important.

In my own case, one way I helped myself to conquer my physical pain was through putting myself on a rigorous exercise schedule of walking. Each week, I would increase the amount I walked by a half mile or more, even though I was afraid I wouldn't be able to make it. Sometimes, it is true, my body gave out on me. But over time, regularly challenging myself to do what I thought I couldn't do played an important role not only in conquering my fear of pain but also in reducing that pain. In fact, I recuperated so completely that eventually I ran fifteen marathons and competed in three triathlons.

Ask yourself if you can mobilize your psychological strength and fighting response to find greater control over your pain. This can be hard when pain is a constant reality in your life, but if you practice long term, it can have very substantial benefits.

RECOMMENDATIONS

Fear of physical pain is a major cause of pain. For people who suffer from chronic pain, learning to challenge the fear of physical pain and to change habitual patterns of worry plays a major role in reducing and sometimes even eliminating that pain.

Each of the four techniques for managing your fear of chronic pain—visualization; breath awareness; nonjudgmental appreciation of body sensations, including sensations of pain; and mobilization of your psychological strength—used regularly and consistently, can have a profound effect on your healing process. Ultimately, these strategies affect the mental and emotional attitudes that dominate your life, moving you out of any fear patterns that may weaken you into greater self-assertion and confidence. The benefits to your body are immediate and reflected in greater vitality and a reduction of pain.

FURTHER READING

Fred Amir, *Rapid Recovery from Back and Neck Pain* (Santa Clara, CA: Health Advisory Group, 1999). Includes an excellent discussion of how fear of pain aggravates pain and conquering fear relieves and eliminates it.

Gerald Epstein, *Healing Visualizations: Creating Health Through Imagery* (New York: Bantam, 1989). A book on the power of imagery for healing by a doctor who trains patients in visualization.

Conclusion

When chronic pain strikes, it's natural to feel somewhat hopeless and helpless. Has anything in your education prepared you to deal with the experience? Perhaps you studied English, mathematics, and the sciences in school, but how much time did you spend studying how your own body works? Or what creates pain? Or how your patterns of movement can make you more or less comfortable and efficient? Or how muscles affect one another? Or how emotions affect your muscles? And how much time did you spend applying knowledge about any of these subjects to exploring your own body?

Chances are that if you are like most people, you have spent close to zero time on these subjects. And so when pain strikes, you may try to ignore it or grin and bear it. If you are lucky, the pain will go away; but it is just as likely that it will get worse over time. You may try to push through the pain, to force your body to work harder to do the things it used to do easily. Inside you are screaming, but you keep on typing away at the computer, even though your shoulders and arms are killing you. Or you keep on lifting weights, trying to make yourself stronger even as it hurts more and more. If you take this approach, your pains will definitely multiply.

Finally, you may try to get someone or something to make the pain go away. You seek an *external* solution to your problem, rather than one that comes from within, from your own explorations of yourself. Now you put your trust in medical specialists. You go to the doctor and get medication. You visit the chiropractor once a week for months or even years. You get hot packs and spinal manipulations from your physical therapist. Or you get a knee or hip replaced or vertebrae fused. All of these options take a lot out of your pocketbook. And sometimes they help. But sometimes they don't. Or they work short term but leave you with bigger problems down the road. Two years after the knee replacement, your hip may need replacement too! Or you end up taking twice the medication you once needed, with less effect on your pain. Meanwhile, your digestive tract is becoming a real problem!

At a deeper level, seeking external solutions to chronic pain problems leaves you disempowered. Here you are, living in your body and asking someone else to fix it. When it comes to chronic pain, this is a very tricky position to be in, because pain is intimately related to stress, and the one thing that creates the most stress in our lives is the feeling of being disempowered and out of control.

The preceding chapters give you tools for getting back in control of your body and reducing your pain. Depending on your history, the chances are also good that if you stay with and pursue more deeply the approach outlined here, you may even completely eliminate your pain.

In the end, your history of chronic pain is about your journey into taking charge of your life. What does this mean? First, it means that pain is a whole-body experience. You may feel your pain in a specific location, but that location reflects the intersection of many interacting physical forces throughout your body: your muscles, fascia, and nerves and their relationship to your joints and bones. To reduce pain in a specific location, you have to get in touch with and improve the way your whole body moves, moment by moment and day by day. Your back pain may be the result of the way your feet hit the ground, or of chronic tension patterns in your neck, or of a rigid diaphragm. You have to pay attention to all of you, be present to all of your body, to undo what is causing your pain. That involves a process of investigation, of being a detective exploring the trail you leave in your life. No one but you can figure out where you hold tension and how to let it go. No one but you can figure out the true causes of your physical pain. Anything else is a poor substitute at best.

Second, pain is not only a whole-body phenomenon, it is also a whole-person phenomenon. Pain is never purely structural or biochemical in origin. It results from a complex dialogue among mental, emotional, and physical aspects of your being, a dialogue whose dynamics have been fleshed out in the chapters on stress and on how stress affects all levels of your being. To reduce chronic pain and to heal yourself is to address your whole person: the way you respond to and relate to life as a whole.

Chronic pain is a pain. There's no doubt about that. But it is also a fabulous teaching tool—a tool you can utilize to learn not only how to manage your body better but also how to be increasingly present to your life and increasingly empowered—physically, mentally, emotionally, and spiritually.

The techniques in this book will help your physical healing, but they will also lead you down the road of personal empowerment. The more you use these techniques, the more empowered you will be. The more empowered you are, the less likely you will be to experience chronic pain. Finally, the more empowered you are, the more likely you will be to find your life rich and fulfilling. Thank you for taking the time to explore the strategies for taking charge of your life that are described in this book. And enjoy your journey into increasingly good health!

Appendix: Nutrition and Chronic Pain

Early in my work with self-healing, I discovered that nutrition plays an important role in reducing chronic pain. Eliminating processed foods, coffee, and sugar from my diet and eating an organically based diet rich in vegetables, fish, and free-range meats contributed significantly to my recovery. Over the years, I have pursued my amateur interest in nutrition, reading widely, testing different dietary approaches, and seeking out experts in the field. In 2001, I met and began working with a clinical nutritionist, Dr. Maile Pouls, who has worked with thousands of clients and written extensively on the relationship between chronic pain and nutrition. In the years that I have known her, I have both benefited personally from her nutritional recommendations and seen many of my clients benefit from them.

Each person's nutritional needs are unique. From her work with thousands of clients, however, Dr. Pouls has identified nutritional problems and deficiencies that are common to many, if not most, cases of chronic pain, most particularly to cases of pain that involve inflammation or fibromyalgia. You can speed your recovery by addressing these problems.

THE ACID CONNECTION
One common denominator of people suffering from fibromyalgia, inflammation, and pain is a urine acid-to-base ratio (pH) that is acidic

(lower than 6.3). You can buy urine pH test strips to test your own urine at any pharmacy. Acidity does not just manifest in the urine. It spreads through the whole body, creating or contributing to inflammatory, degenerative, and painful conditions. Working to eliminate the acidity of your body and improving your overall digestion will help ease your pain. *Avoid acid foods!* The most acid foods, in order of decreasing acidity, are:

1. *Sugar.* This comprises all sweeteners, including but not limited to white sugar, honey, and maple syrup. Not only does sugar promote acidity in the body, it also has no nutritional value, provides empty calories, and weakens the immune system for up to fourteen hours after ingestion. As alternatives consider Stevia or Xylitol, natural sweeteners that do not affect blood sugar levels.

2. *Coffee.* The roasted oils in coffee make it acidic and very hard on the stomach. Coffee also depletes the adrenal glands, our "stress and shock absorber" glands, contributing to increased stress and fatigue. As an alternative to coffee, consider herbal teas and roasted-grain drinks.

3. *Sodas and all carbonated drinks.* Carbonated drinks acidify the body and leach calcium out of the bones. Sodas are also dehydrating, and dehydration contributes to pain. One soda may contain up to ten teaspoons of sugar, which is highly acidifying. Diet sodas are also toxifying.

4. *Alcohol.* Alcohol is very acidic and very high in sugars, and, because it is hard on the liver, it negatively impacts the entire digestive process.

5. *Highly processed and packaged foods.* These are all acidic. Try to eat foods that are as close to "live" as possible. Avoid foods with chemical additives and hydrogenated oils.

6. *Red meats.* Commercially raised animals are given numerous growth enhancers, hormones, and antibiotics, all of which contribute to toxicity and acidity in the consumer's body. If you eat red meat, try to eat organic. Try also to replace some red meat with free-range,

preferably organic poultry, since factory-farmed chickens are fed all kinds of chemicals. Consider eating more fresh cold-water fish.

Replace acidifying foods with alkalinizing foods. The most alkalinizing foods are vegetables (except tomatoes); the darker and greener they are, the more alkaline they are. Eat a variety of organic vegetables that are rich in color. Ask your local supermarket to stock organic vegetables, fruits, and meats.

If you consume dairy products, try to buy only organic butter, milk, and cheese. Commercial dairy products can be loaded with human-made chemicals, hormones, growth promoters, antibiotics, veterinary drugs, and traces of herbicides and pesticides.

Drink plenty of water. Most people do not. Dehydration is a primary cause of muscle and joint pain. To determine the correct amount of water for you, divide your weight in pounds by two. This equals the number of ounces of water you should drink *every day*. Keep a record of how much you drink, and see if you are consuming enough water.

Consider taking supplemental digestive enzymes to improve your digestion. Specific enzymes can reduce fermentation, putrefaction, and acid created throughout the gastrointestinal tract. Take a liver support supplement, in the form of milk thistle or artichoke, to gently detoxify your body of chemicals, heavy metals, and toxins that increase pain and inflammation. Finally, consider cleansing your body through colon cleanses or by taking fiber, in the form of psyllium husks and powder, to regulate your bowel movements and detoxify your colon.

NUTRITIONAL DEFICIENCIES

People suffering from chronic pain, fibromyalgia, and inflammation tend to have common nutritional deficiencies. These include:

1. *Calcium and magnesium.* These minerals are essential for proper muscle and nerve function and need to be balanced in the

body. Magnesium levels frequently decline as we age, contributing to restless leg syndrome, cramping, and sudden muscle spasms. Consider taking a calcium/magnesium supplement. The combination of magnesium and malic acid seems to be particularly helpful in improving the ability of people with pain to exercise, to recover from exercise, and to maintain their activities of daily living.

2. *Electrolytes and trace minerals.* Many people are deficient in trace minerals. Our body depends for its trace minerals on a diet rich in organic vegetables and fruits, something many people lack. Liquid ionic minerals can help maintain the health of all the cells and tissues of the body while reducing spasms and tissue pain.

3. *Essential fatty acids.* Omega-3 essential fatty acids are very effective for decreasing inflammation and pain. They can be consumed in capsule form or taken nutritionally. Nutritional sources of omega-3 essential fatty acids include flaxseed oil and fish oils. In addition, each day add one to two tablespoons of ground flax seeds to salads, fruits, smoothies, and any other noncooked foods with which they go well.

While most omega-6—in contrast to omega-3—essential fatty acids are proinflammatory, there are two notable exceptions: borage oil and evening primrose oil can be extremely beneficial in reducing inflammation.

4. *Vitamin C and other antioxidants.* Antioxidants help reduce inflammation in the body by quenching free radicals and reducing oxidation in the body.

5. *Plant-based digestive enzymes.* Due to years of eating cooked and processed foods, up to 95 percent of the U.S. population is deficient in digestive enzymes. This creates a problem of poor digestion, which contributes to acid conditions and nutrient deficiencies. Digestive enzyme supplementation is vital for the utilization of nutrients from your diet and supplements. In addition, specific plant-based enzymes, such as bromelain and protease enzymes, help reduce inflammation, swelling, redness, and pain.

6. *B vitamins, adaptogenic herbs, and organic adrenal glandulars.* These supplements all promote the body's ability to deal with the nutritionally destructive consequences of stress.

TAKING CHARGE OF YOUR SPECIFIC NUTRITIONAL NEEDS

By following the dietary recommendations above and including the recommended supplements in your diet, you will go a long way toward creating the digestive basis for a healthier body. Each person, however, has a unique nutritional history and unique needs related to his or her lifestyle, diet, stress factors, and genetic predisposition. You may wish to consult a clinical nutritionist who can help you determine your body's specific individual needs.

Dr. Pouls evaluates her patients long distance, through a combination of in-depth diet and health histories, and a biochemical diagnostic evaluation performed on a twenty-four-hour urine sample. Each patient receives an hour-long initial phone consultation subsequent to Dr. Pouls's receipt via the mail of urine samples and health histories. Consultation includes detailed dietary recommendations, explanations of underlying nutritional imbalances, and recommendations for specific supplements to nourish, repair, and rebalance the body, thus addressing many underlying root causes that produce pain and degeneration. Colon, liver, or lymphatic cleansing and detoxification are also encouraged when necessary. If you wish to consider consulting with Dr. Pouls, you can call her toll-free number at 1-877-688-7426 (1-877-NUTRICO).

Products by Ingrid Bacci

VIDEO OR DVD

"Reduce Your Chronic Pain." This 2¼-hour video/DVD, hosted and demonstrated by Ingrid Bacci, presents techniques for self-healing from chronic pain. It includes detailed audiovisual guidance through the following movement patterns: (1) "Improve Your Alignment When Sitting," chapter 7; (2) "Improve Your Alignment When Walking," chapter 7; (3) "Roll Over; Move like a Baby," chapter 9; (4) "The Pelvic Tilt," chapter 9; (5) "Move like a Cat—with Flow," chapter 9.

AUDIOCASSETTES OR CDs

1. *"Breath Awareness" audiocassette/CD.* This audiocassette/CD presents two twenty-minute breath awareness exercises that are excellent for pain and stress reduction. Side 1 offers a meditative breathing exercise ("Meditative Breathing," chapter 5). Side 2 guides you through learning how to be present to relaxed breathing in daily activities. Narrated by Ingrid Bacci, with gentle musical background accompaniment.

2. *"Body Awareness" audiocassette/CD.* This audiocassette/CD presents two twenty-minute exercises to enhance bodily relaxation and tension release. Side 1 offers a body scan ("Body Scan," chapter 9).

Side 2 takes the listener through releasing body tension during activities. Narrated by Ingrid Bacci, with gentle musical background accompaniment.

3. *"Visualization" audiocassette*/CD. This audiocassette/CD presents three fifteen-minute exercises that assist the listener in developing the skills of visualization discussed in chapter 15 on conquering fear of pain. Narrated by Ingrid Bacci, with gentle musical background accompaniment.

To order any products, please go to www.ingridbacci.com.

Index

About the Author

INGRID BACCI, PH.D., C.S.T., CAT, is a complementary health care practitioner, and a consultant to corporations, health maintenance organizations, and hospitals. She is a licensed Alexander Technique teacher and a certified craniosacral therapist. Dr. Bacci teaches seminars on chronic pain management and stress reduction for the HMO Oxford Health Plans, offers training programs in craniosacral therapy on a national level through the Upledger Institute, and is an occasional guest lecturer at the Columbia College of Physicians and Surgeons.

Dr. Bacci specializes in teaching clients how to use self-awareness techniques to overcome chronic pain and stress. Her expertise grew out of her own experiences recovering from a crippling musculoskeletal condition (fibromyalgia) that kept her bedridden for three years. A graduate of Harvard and Columbia universities and a young professor at the time, she left her career to explore complementary healing modalities after prolonged medication and hospital care failed to improve her situation. As a result of her complete recovery, her extensive training in various forms of bodywork, and her work with clients over twenty years, Dr. Bacci has developed a system of body-centered tools for helping individuals achieve freedom from pain and enhanced vitality. Aspects of this system are mapped out in her first book, *The Art of Effortless Living* (Perigee, June 2002), which received high acclaim from recognized authors in the fields of the health and healing.

Dr. Bacci's private practice also incorporates extensive use of the Alexander Technique and other movement awareness techniques, of breathing techniques, and of craniosacral therapy, a soft-touch, scientifically based hands-on therapy that can be highly effective in reducing chronic pain.

THE ART OF EFFORTLESS LIVING
Simple techniques for Healing Mind, Body and Spirit
by Ingrid Bacci Ph.D.

'A profound and potent guide to making transformative shifts in
body, mind and spirit'
Jean Houston, Ph.D., author of *The Search for the Beloved*

Most of us believe that in order to achieve anything worthwhile,
whether in our careers, family life, health or even on the sports
field, we have to work hard and apply a lot of effort. In fact, just the
opposite is true. In *The Art of Effortless Living*, Dr Ingrid Bacci
offers compelling evidence that the most productive, creative and
healthiest individuals are those who practice effortless living. By
doing less, paradoxical as it may seem, they achieve more.

Here, as you learn how to dissolve conscious and unconscious stress
through simple techniques that replace effort with effortlessness,
you will discover a more rewarding lifestyle that leads to physical
vitality, increased productivity, creative relationships and the
freedom to express your best self.

'This book contains a piece of essential wisdom – that by letting go
we gain more, not less. Because most of us are obsessed with the
idea of making things happen, we seriously need the lessons of *The
Art of Effortless Living*'
Larry Dossey, M.D., author of *Recovering Your Soul*

0 553 81440 0

BANTAM BOOKS

PERFECT HEALTH
by Deepak Chopra

'A brilliant and exhilarating book'
Sunday Telegraph

A decade ago, Deepak Chopra, M.D., wrote the international
bestseller, *Perfect Health*, the first practical guide to harnessing the
healing power of the mind. Describing how breakthroughs in physics
and medicine were underscoring the validity of a 5,000-year-old
medical system from India known as Ayurveda, it went on to reveal
how this ancient wisdom could be applied to everyday life, Now, in
celebration of this classic work, this new edition has been revised and
updated to include the very latest medical research.

Although we experience our bodies as solid, they are in fact more
like fires that are constantly being consumed and renewed. We grow
new stomach linings every five days, for instance; our skin is new every
five weeks; each year, ninety-eight per cent of the total number of
atoms in our bodies is replaced. Ayurveda gives us the tools to
intervene at this quantum level, where we are being created anew
each day. It also reveals how freedom from sickness depends on
contacting our own awareness, bringing it into balance and then
extending that balance to the body.

Perfect Health provides a complete step-by-step programme of
mind-body medicine tailored to individual needs. A quiz identifies
the reader's mind-body type: thin, restless Vata; enterprising, efficient
Pitta; tranquil, steady Kapha: or any combination of these three.
It is this body type that forms the basis of a specific Ayurvedic
programme of diet, stress reduction, neuromuscular integration,
exercise, and daily routines. The result is a total health plan that
will re-establish the body's essential balance with nature, strengthen
the mind-body connection, and use the power of quantum healing
to transcend the ordinary limitations of disease and aging. In short,
this is the ultimate guide to achieving Perfect Health.

DEEPAK CHOPRA has written twenty-six books, including the
international bestseller *The Seven Spiritual Laws of Success*. In 1999,
Time Magazine selected Dr. Chopra as one of the Top 100 Icons
and Heroes of the Century, describing him as 'the poet-prophet of
alternative medicine'. He currently serves as CEO and founder of
The Chopra Center for Well Being in La Jolla, California.

0 553 81367 6

BANTAM BOOKS